Silent Crusader

*How One Woman's Struggles
Changed Many Lives*

Cheryl Kantak

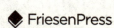
FriesenPress

One Printers Way
Altona, MB R0G 0B0
Canada

www.friesenpress.com

Copyright © 2023 by Cheryl Kantak
First Edition — 2023

All rights reserved.

No part of this publication may be reproduced in any form, or by any means, electronic or mechanical, including photocopying, recording, or any information browsing, storage, or retrieval system, without permission in writing from FriesenPress.

ISBN
978-1-03-918596-8 (Hardcover)
978-1-03-918595-1 (Paperback)
978-1-03-918597-5 (eBook)

1. BIOGRAPHY & AUTOBIOGRAPHY, PERSONAL MEMOIRS

Distributed to the trade by The Ingram Book Company

Silent Crusader

*How One Woman's Struggles
Changed Many Lives*

TABLE OF CONTENTS

Introduction   1

CHAPTER 1
Starting Our Family   3

CHAPTER 2
Making an Impact   31

CHAPTER 3
Problems, Questions, and Discoveries   39

CHAPTER 4
Formal Education Begins   57

CHAPTER 5
The School for the Deaf   73

CHAPTER 6
Cindy Attends Our Local High School   95

CHAPTER 7
The Fight Took Its Toll; Cindy Moves Out   125

CHAPTER 8
Facilitated Communication   141

CHAPTER 9
We Fight for Cindy   159

CHAPTER 10
The State Insists on Keeping Control **183**

CHAPTER 11
More Problems and Changes Cause Us to Rethink Our Plan **201**

CHAPTER 12
How Are the Girls Doing Now? **219**

Final Thoughts and Acknowledgements **225**

Dedications

For Cindy and Deb
My beautiful daughters who have inspired me, taught me so much, and brought us immeasurable joy

For Bob
Thanks for being there for me. I love you

For Scott
The best brother anyone could have

And for all the parents and family members of individuals with disabilities who deal with these issues and so much more

Introduction

This is a story about my daughter, Cynthia. Cindy lives in her own home with support provided in various ways twenty-four hours a day. Cindy is extremely happy and maintains a busy lifestyle. She enjoys swimming, horseback riding, drawing on the computer, craft projects, and painting. She loves to travel and dine out, and is definitely a party girl. Cindy enjoys being around other people, and they also enjoy her company. Cindy's life has impacted so many others. She has touched the hearts of so many people and taught them the meaning of courage and strength. She has shown over and over what it means to not give up. She has been a pioneer of changes paving the way so others may have an easier time. She has had many struggles, but through them all, she has been a true champion, intent and passionate about life. She has faced her challenges with zeal and enthusiasm. Although she cannot speak, her voice has been heard loud and its echo has resonated. Many people have been influenced by Cindy and have benefited from all she has accomplished. I hope I can give you just a piece of that in her story.

Most of the names and places have been changed. Some have not. But the story is true as I remember it. The feelings and emotions expressed are very real. Some things you never forget.

Chapter 1
STARTING OUR FAMILY

Bob and I were married in the fall of 1968 in Syracuse, New York, where we both grew up. He was twenty-six years old, and I was twenty-two. We both had full-time jobs. Bob worked for the local utility company, and I worked for an airline. We enjoyed a busy, active life that included among other things social outings with friends, sporting events, and vacations.

In the summer of 1971 when I became pregnant with Cindy, I was filled with so many mixed emotions. Bob was thrilled and received the news with great anticipation. I was happy, of course, but also very fearful. I was afraid I would not be a good mother, probably a natural reaction. But I was also afraid of losing my freedom, my career, and my identity. I loved my current job as an insurance underwriter and I was very good at it. I had worked my way up to be the supervisor of the department and I was proud of what I had accomplished. I did not want to give that up.

I also had another very strong fear. Because I was adopted and knew nothing about my biological parents, I was anxious about what I would be passing down. When I was a young child, I accidentally overheard a conversation and learned I was adopted. When I asked about it, my mother told me several different stories. First, she said that my parents were married and loved me and wanted me very much but could not afford to raise a child. Even as young as I was, somehow that did not seem right to me. I felt there had to be another reason. Sometimes, when I would question my mother, the story would change, and she always seemed nervous when answering. I convinced myself that there was something awful she was hiding.

When I was in high school, I approached the subject again; my mother confessed that I was born out of wedlock. I was incredibly relieved; that made sense to me and I accepted it. But for some reason, I could not rid myself of the fear of what I would pass down or what the baby would look like. My mother tried to ease my anxiety. She assured me that my birth mother was a young healthy woman in her late teens or early twenties who just happened to get in trouble. My mother told me she spoke directly to the attorney who met the girl when the adoption was finalized. He reassured my mother I had nothing to worry about. But there was no information about the father, and whatever my mother said did little to ease my fears. Perhaps it was all the years I spent thinking there was a horrible secret.

Although it would not have helped me through that difficult time, I did register with the New York State Adoption Registry many years later. I did not find out much but I did learn that my biological mother was 35 years old and unmarried at the time of my birth. The knowledge I gained only intensified my fears. As I look back on it now, I realize that the kinds of things I worried about then were selfish and entirely the wrong things, but at the time they seemed very important. I never gave a thought to the possibility that something could be physically wrong with the baby. In my mind, that only happened to other people. Ironically, many years later, I would learn I inherited a neurological disease from my mother.

MY PREGNANCY

I had a difficult pregnancy to say the least. My problems started at four and a half months when I started bleeding. Bob rushed me to the ER, and I was subsequently admitted to the hospital; the doctors thought I was going to miscarry. I was given a shot and put on bed rest. A few days later, when nothing else happened, I was released and told to go home and take it easy. I took sick leave from my job. Unfortunately, the bleeding happened again a few weeks later, and I was again hospitalized. When I was sent home several days later, I was put on total bed rest for the remainder of my pregnancy. At six months, I started bleeding heavily again. Bob was bowling in a tournament when it started, and I had to call him away in the middle of a match. My brother-in-law drove me to the hospital, and Bob met me there. This scenario would repeat itself as I ended up going to the hospital five times.

At seven months, my water broke and the doctors were sure I was going to go into labor, so they sent me to the labor and delivery unit. Bob and I were so afraid. X-rays were taken and we were told as far as they could tell everything was all right. There was a huge snowstorm that night, and Bob ended up sleeping on the floor of the labor room next to me. Eventually, the doctors decided I was not going to go into labor. They put me back on the maternity ward where I stayed for two weeks before returning home again on total bed rest. Cindy was a fighter even before she was born. My pregnancy was obviously not a pleasant one as I bled consistently throughout it, and the last six weeks, I had to wear adult diapers because my membranes had ruptured and I was still creating amniotic fluid.

Eventually, I was hospitalized again to determine whether a Caesarian section should be done. I had several more tests along the way, including X-rays, and was told everything looked OK. The doctors, however, were very worried about whether the baby's lungs were developed enough. So even though it was very late in the pregnancy, I also had an amniocentesis. I had no knowledge of this test, and the procedure was explained to me. Because my membranes had already ruptured, getting sufficient amniotic fluid was difficult. I was told the result showed that the lungs were developed enough, and they would do the Caesarian and take the baby early.

Because I was so anemic, it was necessary to give me a blood transfusion before the surgery. While receiving that transfusion, the night before the scheduled procedure, I went into labor. I was vomiting and had pains that were so mild that the nurses and doctors were disagreeing on whether I was really in labor. About 11:00 that night, a doctor came and examined me and ordered that I go to the labor and delivery unit. I was transferred to that unit, and my husband was told to go home and come back the next day, as I would be in labor for a long time. He hung around for a while and finally left about 1:30 a.m. He no sooner got home then he received a call that I was going into delivery. He rushed right back. Cindy was born about 2:30 a.m.

I was surprised I had gone into delivery so soon, as I had expected to have hours and hours of screaming with pain. I had arranged long before to have a spinal because I had been so afraid of the actual birthing process, but the spinal was worse than the labor. I do not know why they decided to give it to me but I did not argue. At that point in time, I was just so glad it was all finally over. Little did I know it was only the beginning.

When Cindy was delivered, I was told we had a girl. I remember there seemed to be a flurry of activity but I really did not think too much of it. I also did not think at that time that it was strange they did not show her to me immediately. My obstetrician came over to finish with me, and I asked if she was OK. He said her foot was a little turned but that could be fixed. They very briefly showed her to me from across the room, and I was wheeled out of the delivery room to where my husband, Bob, was standing right outside the door waiting.

"Well, you didn't get your boy," I spoke.

"I didn't? What did I get?" he replied.

"By process of elimination I think it is a girl." We both laughed. Her name was Cynthia Anne; we had picked out both a boy's and girl's name prior to the delivery. We both went into recovery where we spent a few joyous moments.

NOT WHAT WE EXPECTED

My obstetrician had prearranged for a pediatrician to be on hand "just in case." We had spoken to him on the phone weeks before, and he assured me it was just a precaution. A few minutes after arriving in recovery, a man walked into the room and introduced himself as Dr. Schaffer, the one I had spoken to on the phone. He was one of three doctors in the pediatric firm. He suggested that my husband sit down.

"I can tell you the least that is wrong with your daughter." I remember those words like they were spoken yesterday. I remember the rest of what he said but not necessarily the exact words. He seemed to go on forever.

"Her esophagus is not connected to her stomach, so she can't be fed by mouth.[1] Her nose is totally blocked by bone, so she cannot breathe through her nose.[2] Because babies naturally do that, we have had to put a mouthpiece in to keep her mouth open. There are serious problems with her heart, and we don't know the full extent of it as yet. We will have to call in a specialist. We know there is a hole between the chambers.[3] She is missing her right tibia, which is the major bone in the lower leg. Her right leg is short and the foot

---

1 Tracheoesophageal fistula
2 Choanal atresia
3 Ventricular septal defect

deformed and it has an extra digit. She also has an extra digit on her left hand.[4] An orthopedic specialist will need to look at her. Her survival is questionable, and she will be immediately transferred by ambulance to another hospital, which has an intensive care unit." He asked my husband if he had seen his daughter yet and was told no. He then excused himself and said he would be back.

That time is so vivid in my memory yet so foggy. Bob told me many years later that he looked at me and saw that every part of me that was exposed was deep red except for my forehead, which was stark white. I began to cry, and Bob consoled me as best he could. A nurse came in and poured a cup of water and handed me a huge pill. When I asked what it was, she coldly said, "It is to dry up your milk as there won't be any breastfeeding now." I think I began to cry even harder and was then told by her to stop it because it wasn't going to do any good. Eventually, I believe they gave me a tranquilizer to calm me down.

Dr. Schaffer came back in and said the arrangements had been made for the ambulance and told my husband to come with him so he could see his daughter. I asked to see her before she left. Bob was gone only a short time and when he came back, he told me that Cindy had been baptized by one of the nurses as her condition was critical. A short while later, two very nice male attendants came in pushing a gurney that carried our daughter inside an isolette. With them was a lovely nurse who said she would accompany Cindy during the transfer. They all assured us they would take good care of her. I got a brief look at Cindy. She was swaddled in a blanket and had a mouthpiece. Although she looked very small, she was beautiful. They didn't stay long as getting her to a pediatric ICU was urgent. They were all very

---

4   Polydactyly

kind, compassionate, and understanding, and I think I thanked them. After they left, I cried some more.

I then asked Bob if he had called our parents. It was still very early in the morning, and he told me he thought we should wait a little while. I think I was unaware at the time how difficult that task was for him. I couldn't understand why he kept putting it off. Not only did he have a hysterical wife on his hands while dealing with his own emotions, but he was the one who had to break the news to the rest of the family. It was Bob who ended up having to repeat the bad news over and over and deal with everyone's reactions. He told me much later that when he went to his parents' house to tell them about Cindy, his mother fainted. Then he had to call my parents who were living in Florida at the time and eagerly awaiting news of the arrival of their first grandchild. When he called them, he had great difficulty speaking, yet my mother kept questioning him about the details of what was wrong with the baby. Eventually, she stopped and said they would leave right away. Looking back, I don't know how Bob was able to do everything he did. On second thought, I do know. He did it the same way we both have done so many other difficult things since then — he had no choice. Someone had to tell our family.

Soon after the delivery, I was transferred back to a regular room on the maternity ward. I was provided a private room, not because I requested it but because it was available and I was emotionally a wreck. I remember how difficult it was to be on that floor watching all the babies being wheeled by. There was no baby brought to me, no flowers delivered, no happy smiles or joyous grandparents. Mostly I just cried. One nurse came in to see me and told me to go ahead and cry all I wanted. She said she understood because she had had a similar experience with her own child. I immediately connected with her and began to talk about the many things that were wrong. I mentioned to her about something not being connected to the stomach, unsure of the correct terminology. She responded by asking if the baby had a stomach. I suddenly realized just how critical this really was.

A priest from the church Bob and I attended visited me. My sister-in-law had called him. I think he did the usual kinds of things that they do but I only remember one thing. Bob was there at the time, and the priest looked at us and said, "Don't let this come between the two of you." I had no idea at the time what he meant, but the advice has always stuck in my mind. It was good advice.

Bob went to our church later that day. This was the church he and his entire family had attended for many years. He went to the school associated with it and graduated from the high school. When he got there, the doors were locked. He knocked and someone opened the door and told him the church was closed. He explained the situation and told the person he just wanted to light a candle and say some prayers for Cindy's survival. He was told the church was closed. He was turned away. I can only imagine how alone and abandoned he must have felt. We never heard anything from the church again.

Sometime that first afternoon we received a call from the pediatric cardiologist. He told me that Cindy's heart was on the wrong side or turned around,[5] and there was a problem with the pulmonary artery.[6] They suspected there may be something else wrong, but that couldn't be determined until further tests were completed.

My obstetrician also came to see me. He too was very somber. When he asked if I knew anything about how the baby was, I told him what I knew. I remember he stared out the window almost the entire visit.

"Sometimes doctors question whether or not they have done the right thing," he said. He told me he was a Catholic. I wondered if

---

5   Dextrocardia

6   Pulmonary Stenosis

he thought that perhaps he should not have done so much for me to keep the baby when I was having so much trouble.

"Usually, babies with these kinds of problems don't survive." As he was talking to me, his voice often cracked.

Staying in the hospital was so difficult for me, and I told him I wanted to go home. He said he would be back in the morning and see how I was feeling. Bob spent as much time with me as he could until I and the nurses convinced him to go home and get some rest.

When Bob got home that afternoon, his parents were already at the house and were in the process of cleaning out our linen closet. At the time I couldn't understand why they felt that was important. Bob told me at that point in time he did not want to talk and cleaning the closet was the furthest thing in his mind. He went into our bedroom to lay down. Fortunately, his brother came and went in, and they talked for some time. It was many years later that I realized people handle grief in different ways. Bob's parents didn't know what to do, so I guess they just kept busy and did whatever came to mind. They weren't the only ones. Many people didn't know what to say or do and felt awkward, so they stayed away. Because of that, we never got calls of congratulations or visits from friends bearing gifts. We never heard from most of our family and friends. If we did, it was a message of condolences. The flowers we received had messages of sympathy not congratulations. It was more like a funeral than a birth.

My obstetrician came in the next morning and gave me permission to go home, provided that I rest. I asked if I could stop at the hospital and see Cindy, and after a long hesitation, he said it would be OK. My mother-in-law was with Bob when he picked me up, and we all went to see Cindy. After having to put on a gown and wash our hands, we were allowed in the intensive care nursery. I was led to an incubator and saw Cindy for the second time. I was so weak, and my legs could barely hold me; Bob and his mother held me up. Cindy was beautiful, with a full head of dark brown — almost black — hair except for one side where it had been shaved to insert a tube. She had the biggest, darkest brown eyes; they were almost black. She was naked, with several tubes coming out of her, and I didn't even know what they were all doing. She was so tiny, under five pounds, and I wasn't allowed to hold her, so I reached through the little hole and touched her tiny hand. Then I stroked a part of her head and I swear she knew it was me and she looked my way. She seemed so full of life despite her being so sick. The nurse told me that she was going to have surgery the next day to try to repair her esophagus. I asked if the doctor would call me, and she said that he would.

AT HOME WITH NO BABY

That afternoon at home, I waited for my parents to arrive. They had left Florida to drive up right after Bob called and told them about Cindy. My brother, who lived about an hour and a half away and didn't have an available car, hitched a ride with someone so he could see me. I was always close to my brother, and he was a great comfort to me.

While waiting for my parents, we received a call from the surgeon, Dr. Franco, who told us he had inserted a gastrostomy tube into Cindy's stomach so she could be fed. It was a rubber tube that hung down from her stomach about six or eight inches with a clamp at the end. Formula was put through it using a large syringe and that is how she was fed for well over a year. He told us the procedure went well and that the next day he would be doing the critical and delicate surgery to repair her esophagus. He was kind and soft spoken and very patient with me and assured me he would call the next day.

My parents arrived later that day, and after a while I wanted to take them to the hospital to see Cindy. Bob didn't think it was a good idea and tried to stop me from going. My parents and I went but Bob did not. When we saw Cindy, I noticed how pale my mother looked, and my dad had to leave the room because he was so upset. Now she had even more tubes than before, but she was still beautiful. I felt so weak and emotionally drained, but every time I looked at her and how hard she was fighting, I gained some strength. I remember thinking if someone so small and helpless could fight that hard and be so strong, then I could too. Cindy gave me the strength and courage to go on and not fall apart.

The next day I wanted to go to the hospital again to see Cindy, but Bob talked me out of it. He thought it would be good for me to just get some different scenery so he took me for a ride in the car and we stopped for lunch. What I didn't know at the time is that one of the pediatricians, Dr. Williams, had called Bob at home the day Cindy was born. He told him to try to keep me away from the baby; it was doubtful she would survive, and it would be better if I did not become attached. He further advised that if she did survive, she would have many problems and probably would have to live in an institution. That was why Bob had tried to discourage me from going to the hospital and made the effort to keep me away. He thought he was doing the right thing. I think he realized after that first day that it wasn't going to work and he really didn't want it either. Cindy was our daughter and despite her problems we loved her. We couldn't just abandon her.

After our ride that afternoon, we returned home and received several phone calls. People from my office were calling to see how I was and how the baby was doing. I am not sure how they knew about Cindy's birth, but many were calling to offer their condolences. One person I barely knew called to ask just what the matter was with her, wanting details of her problems. I realized how difficult it must have been earlier for Bob as I told the story over and over. There were no offers of congratulations or floral bouquets, no baby gifts, or cute little stuffed animals. Instead, there were tears and expressions of sympathy and endless questions. What was supposed to be a happy time seemed more like a wake, and in many ways, it was just that. It was the death of the healthy, normal child we had hoped to have.

In the afternoon we received another call from Dr. Franco to report on the surgery to repair Cindy's esophagus. Even though we had never met, he impressed me as a very kind and compassionate man. He was incredibly nice on the phone and told us the surgery went well and that the next few critical days would tell a great deal. He asked if I had any questions and told me to call him at any time if I did.

I finally met him many days later when he was making his rounds and checking on Cindy. I was completely taken aback by him as he was well over six feet tall and had what I thought were enormous hands. I remember wondering how this man with such huge hands could ever operate on my very tiny baby. She could easily be held in one hand. I couldn't imagine anyone trying to repair her esophagus, let alone this gigantic man. He was as nice in person as he was on the phone, and I thought him to be a magician to have accomplished what he did. Or perhaps miracle worker would be a better description for Cindy's survival was miraculous. It was the beginning of a long and positive relationship.

DAILY VISITS

Cindy did much better than anyone expected. Bob's attempts to keep me away from her as suggested lasted only the one day, and he no longer could stay away either. That next day we went to visit her, as we did every day for the next two months until she came home. We had stopped at a store and bought her a stuffed animal that played music and put it in the isolette with her. I would wind it up and play it when I was with her, thinking it would soothe her and help her with the pain she must feel. Doctors had told me when I asked that she was too little to feel pain, but I didn't believe them. She was critical, and I couldn't even hold her. So I would sit by the side of the isolette, stick my hand through the holes, and hold her hand or rub her skin wherever I could, because that was all I had. Although Bob was given some time off, eventually he had to go back to work. As we only had one car, I would drive him to work in the morning and then go immediately to the hospital where I would spend the day until I went to pick him up. We would have dinner at home, and then both of us would go to the hospital in the evening. This would be our routine for the next few months.

We saw so many things in that intensive care nursery, some of which were incredibly difficult. The nurses there were just wonderful. I couldn't understand how they could do what they did without getting attached. But of course, they very often did become attached. I watched the nurses cry when a baby died and celebrate when one went home. I witnessed a feud when the family of one baby asked to have the feedings withheld so the baby would eventually die. The nurses refused, and it was a horrible time. I also watched when that same baby was sent away to an institution unwanted by the family. The nurses all chipped in and bought the baby some clothes, and one of the nurses insisted on traveling there with the baby. They all cried and so did I. I often wondered what happened to that child and thought about how it could have easily been Cindy. I remember the baby was sent somewhere down around Utica, New York, and now wonder if it was the Rome Developmental Center, a New York State–run institution for those with disabilities. I didn't know about those kinds of institutions back then.

I finally got to hold Cindy when she was ten days old. It was a wonderful time for me, although I was so frightened I would hurt her. It was difficult as she was hooked up to several tubes. But at least I got to hold her for a short time and I treasured every minute of it.

ANOTHER SHOCK

During those first few days and weeks, we learned the extent of Cindy's heart problems. Her heart was turned around or, as some refer to it, on the wrong side, which is called dextrocardia. She also had pulmonary stenosis, a thickening of the pulmonary artery wall, and a ventricular septal defect, which is a hole in the wall between the chambers of the heart. It was also possible she had what was called tetralogy of fallot,[7] but that wasn't known for sure. It remained to be seen how serious the heart problems were and what other vital organs would be affected. Of course, there was also the problem with her foot, which was noticeably turned. Her right leg did not look right as it was in a bent position and appeared to be too short. But everyone assured me they could "do so much these days," and there were so many other critical things to think about that I shouldn't worry at all about the leg. I believed what people told me, and I really didn't think too much about it.

When Cindy was a few weeks old, I was sitting next to her holding her hand through the porthole of the isolette. I knew an orthopedic doctor was supposed to have come in for a consultation. I asked a nurse if the doctor had been in to see her, and she replied that he had. I asked what he found, and she in turn asked me, "Didn't the doctor call you?" I told her no and continued to question her as to what he said, and she kept telling me that I would have to speak with the doctor. Shortly thereafter, the pediatrician, Dr. Schaffer, came in. He had intended to stop quickly to do something with some charts when the nurse told him I wanted to speak with him. Cindy's isolette was right next to the door, so he stood right outside it and poked his head around so he wouldn't have to go through

---

[7] The combination of four abnormalities of the heart: ventricular septal defect, pulmonary stenosis, hypertrophy of right ventricle, and overriding aorta

the ritual of the dressing gown and so on. He jokingly commented about me holding hands with Cindy, to which I replied it was all I had. I asked what the orthopedic doctor said.

"Oh, just as we suspected, amputation of the lower limbs." Then he turned and left.

I was in total shock. He may have suspected it, but I sure didn't. The nurse must have overheard this because she came right over to me and put her arm around me and asked if I would like to go to the nurse's lounge. I shook my head no and said I had to leave. She tried to get me to stay, but I felt this sense of panic coming over me and I knew I had to get out of there. I told Cindy I loved her and I would be back. I don't know how I managed to safely drive home but I do remember that I kept repeating to myself to concentrate on driving and getting home.

When I arrived home, I picked up the phone and called my sister-in-law. I asked her to have Bob's brother pick him up at work and to please not ask me any questions. She tried to find out what was wrong, and I told her I didn't want to talk about it. She finally just did as I asked. I hung up the phone and went to pieces. I was still sobbing when Bob got home from work, worried about what was going on. After I told him, we both held each other and cried together. At the time, we thought this was the most horrible thing that could happen, and in my despair, I very briefly wondered if it would have been better if she had not survived. Once more, we had to relay this awful news to family and friends and repeat it over and over.

There were many times when I thought I couldn't take any of it anymore. But, every time I looked at Cindy and how hard she was fighting, I thought to myself, if she can do it so can I. She was so small and sick yet she was so strong in spirit. She truly defied all the doctors' predictions. She continued to improve, and in the weeks to come, the nurses would make mention of taking her home. I told them I didn't know how I could do that. I hadn't even changed a diaper before, let alone feed someone through a tube. They assured me they would teach me and that I could do it. So, by sticking my hands through the holes of the isolette, I changed my first diaper. Boy, was I shaking. Soon they taught me how to feed her using the tube.

When she was about six weeks old, Cindy was moved to a regular nursery unit and removed from the isolette. We were thrilled she was doing so well but were struck by the difference in the two units. The pediatric unit Cindy was in had children of all ages, and some would wander around unsupervised. I saw one child playing with the buttons on a baby's isolette and reported it to a nurse. It was the first time I had to report something like that but it definitely was not the last.

Cindy had to have more surgery, this time on her nose. It was totally blocked by bone, called choanal atresia, so the blockage would be drilled opened and a u-shaped tube inserted to keep it open so she could breathe through her nose. The tube would have to be carefully suctioned out with a machine. Bob took time off from work so he could be with me while we waited to hear how the operation went. We waited in the special room and we were relieved when the doctor came and told us the operation went well and she was doing fine. He said she was in recovery and would be up in about thirty minutes. After a while, Bob had to get back to work so he left. I waited and waited and kept checking with the nurses to see if they had heard anything but they had not. I think it was well over an hour and a half before they brought her back. A doctor came over to me.

"Were you on any antibiotics when you were pregnant?" he asked.

"Yes, the last six weeks of the pregnancy I was on ampicillin to prevent infection."

"Oh, then you are at fault," he said half-laughingly. He went on to say that they had given Cindy penicillin, and she had a reaction but they didn't understand why. He further explained that in order to have a reaction, you have to have had the medicine previously, and there was no record of anyone ever giving it to her. So now I was to blame. As if I didn't have enough to deal with, now the doctors were blaming me for Cindy's allergy.

For the next few weeks, Cindy continued to do well, she was tolerating her formula, and there was talk of sending her home. I was so excited that she would finally be coming home but so frightened about all the medical issues I had to deal with. By this time, we were attempting to do some bottle feeding but still needed to use the feeding tube. The hospital arranged for me to have a rented suction machine at home, and they would send home plenty of tubes, syringes, and whatever else we needed. I was scared but also thrilled. Cindy was now two months old and she was finally coming home.

PREPARING FOR CINDY TO COME HOME

Bob and I spent two days doing all the preparations that had not been done previously. Bob put the crib together, and we went out and bought diapers and formula and even some clothes. There had been no baby shower or birth gifts, so we had to get a lot of things. The afternoon before Cindy was to be released, we were shopping for supplies when I started having an upset feeling in my stomach. I told Bob I thought I was going to throw up. We went home and he took my temperature, which was normal. We were worried I was coming down with a stomach bug so we called the hospital and said we would not be up that night and we would see how I felt the next day. Bob called his parents and told them. His father brought me a pill and insisted I take it. I didn't know at the time what it was but I trusted his judgment. It seemed to do the trick as I felt much better relatively quickly. I found out later that he gave me a mild tranquillizer. I didn't have a stomach bug but instead a huge case of the nerves. I guess I was entitled to that and when I realized what it was, I learned to deal with it.

Before Cindy was discharged from the hospital, one of the doctors commented that when she had been in the operating room, they should have taken off the extra digit on her hand but they did not think of it. So they decided to do it the day she came home by tying it off. They told me they would tie a string around it tightly and eventually it would turn black and fall off. They assured me it was better to do it that way. At that time in my life, I believed much of what doctors told me.

AT LAST, CINDY COMES HOME

So we brought Cindy home with all the tubes and machines and medical issues. She was a good baby and seldom cried, except when something was being done to her that was unpleasant. She had to have the tubes in her nose suctioned out as well as her throat, which had a great deal of mucus all the time. Many times, when she was fed through the tube or by bottle, the formula would come back up, and sometimes she would gag. This was something we would go through for many years, even long after the tubes were out. Her esophagus had a great deal of scar tissue and did not expand and contract normally. Food of any kind would become easily stuck, and she would seem to be choking. For many years she would throw up at almost every meal until she learned how to chew her food enough to handle it. Mealtime was always very stressful for us.

The first few weeks after Cindy came home was an especially difficult time for me. It was all still new and scary, and I felt so ill prepared. To make matters worse, the doctor who tied off the extra finger apparently didn't tie it tight enough, and it was not falling off as predicted. It had started to turn black but still had enough blood supply that it wouldn't fall off. I had to change the bandage frequently and when I did, Cindy would scream because it would stick to the site. It was so awful to see and I felt helpless. Bob helped me as much as he could when he was not working, but basically, I was alone. There was a public health nurse who came to see me and check on Cindy once every two weeks for about a half-hour, but most of our time together I spent crying. In those days, there just weren't the kinds of services available to parents that there are today.

Despite all the medical issues, Cindy was a very good-natured baby. Apart from when something was being done to her, she seldom cried. We held her and enjoyed her as any parent would. She already had a happy, good nature. We were thrilled she was finally home with us.

BACK TO THE HOSPITAL

Within the first few weeks of when she came home, she started having problems swallowing and handling her formula. We had to take her to the emergency room. She was admitted to the hospital as her esophagus was closing and she needed to have it dilated. It would be the first of several she would have to have done. I always stayed with her when she was in the hospital as much as I could and I always made sure all the doctors and nurses knew everything there was to know about her. She was scheduled for surgery the next day.

I left her briefly to go get something to eat in the cafeteria. When I came back, she seemed different to me. She seemed to be wheezing more.

"Cindy is not acting right. I think something is wrong," I told a nurse.

She said she would ask a doctor to look at her. I think she thought I was an overreactive parent who didn't know much. No one came to look at her, and I became increasingly alarmed. I kept insisting that a doctor see her immediately. The nurses were becoming more impatient with me but continued to assure me the doctor on call would see her. The doctor on call did pop his head in briefly, but when I told him I thought something was wrong, he shrugged it off and said he would check her out later.

Hours later I became even more upset. I called her ear, nose, and throat doctor and demanded he send someone up to check on Cindy. He did and they found that apparently when I was out of the room someone had suctioned Cindy's nose and either didn't know she had a tube in it or was just careless. They had pushed the tube back down into her throat and she was choking on it. The doctor immediately pulled the tube out completely, and she was no longer in distress. This was one of the many times Cindy taught me to rely on what she was doing and what I knew about her and not what medical professionals told me.

The problem was rectified but I was furious. I went to the nurse's station and asked to see the doctor who was on call and had so quickly popped in. He appeared at the desk and I immediately confronted him.

"Do you have any idea what you have put us through? My daughter could have choked to death."

"I am very busy and she is not my only patient," he said with an arrogant and cocky attitude. He offered no apology.

"If you can't handle the pressure, you better get out of the profession," I screamed. There were many people staring at us, and I thought I was probably the talk of the ward. I really didn't care.

The next day our pediatrician came in to see Cindy, and he said to me that he had heard I had had quite a day. I asked if it was all over the hospital, and he laughed and said no, just the eighth floor. Then he went on to say that perhaps my method wasn't entirely professional but he sure didn't blame me. I really didn't care if it was professional. I was a parent and all I cared about was Cindy getting good care and I had realized it was going to be up to me to make sure she got it. I also learned that even small sick babies have ways of communicating if you know how to look for them. From that day forward, when Cindy was in the hospital, either Bob or I spent as much time as we possibly could with her, even taking shifts overnight. Being so assertive was something very new and different and not always easy for me, but Cindy had taught me that I needed to do it. Cindy gave me strength and confidence.

Cindy had her esophagus dilated and the tube in her nose properly reinserted. While she was under general anesthesia, they also removed the extra digit that was improperly tied off. She remained in the hospital for a few more weeks, and we were back to the daily routine of visiting.

DIFFICULT DECISIONS

When Cindy was three months old, she was again released from the hospital. She was still having a great deal of trouble feeding by mouth and still had all the tubes but she was really progressing nicely. Because she had many doctor appointments and required so much care, I was not able to return to work as I had planned. I was fortunate enough to work for a wonderful company, and the bosses were very understanding. I had held a supervisory position, chief underwriter, when I went on medical leave, and they were holding it open for me. After Cindy's birth, when it became obvious I could not come back on a full-time basis, they eventually filled that position. But they wanted to keep me, and for many months, they allowed me to work at home whenever I could. They even brought the work to me and picked it up. I did work whenever I could, and it was a good distraction. I was good at my job, enjoyed it, and missed it.

I spent most of my time caring for Cindy and shuttling her to doctors. Bob bought a used second car so I would not have to take him back and forth to work. Bob's dad was also wonderful about driving me and Cindy to appointments.

We began meeting with the orthopedic surgeon to discuss our options regarding Cindy's leg. He explained that her foot was really of no use to her as her leg was so much shorter. That would have to be amputated so she could be fitted with a prosthesis. After that we had a choice. He explained that she was missing the right tibia as well as her kneecap and that the lower part of her leg was badly constricted. He wanted to try the "Brown Procedure," named after the doctor who first did it. He would take the remaining bone in her lower leg, the fibula, and center it below the thigh bone or the femur. He would straighten it surgically as much as possible and then later cast it. If successful, she would be fitted with only an artificial foot. The alternative would be to amputate above the knee, in which case she would need a full leg prosthesis. Bob and I agonized over this decision. The doctor told us there was a 50/50 chance the procedure to save the lower part of her leg would be successful, and if it was, she would be much better off. He told us it was always better to keep as much of the limb as possible. We thought the odds for success were good and it might be worth the chance.

Coincidentally, at the time we were discussing this, there was a doctor visiting the hospital from the Midwest. He was apparently very well-known as he was giving many talks. Our doctor asked us if they could present Cindy to him in what they called grand rounds. It was an auditorium full of doctors; I brought Cindy in, and her doctor presented her case and what he wanted to do. The expert gave his opinion that it probably would not work. After that, we met with our doctor again and he still felt she had a good chance. It was very difficult to make this decision, but we had confidence in our orthopedic doctor. I remember Bob and I talking about it and saying to each other that if the decision turned out to be wrong, then at least we knew we did not take it lightly and we did our homework. Someday we would be able to tell Cindy how and why we came to our decision. Of course, we thought we were doing the right thing, but it turned out to be the single worst decision of our life. We were still very naïve and trusting when it came to doctors, and this one charmed us.

THE DOCTORS LEARN FROM CINDY

When she was eight months old, Cindy was hospitalized again to have the first of many orthopedic surgeries. The first surgery (Brown Procedure) was performed to put her fibula underneath the femur, and pins were inserted through the knee area. She was in a cast and would be for several weeks. The surgery supposedly went well, and Cindy was released a few days later.

Shortly after she came home, Cindy started acting like she was in distress. She was not her usual self, instead crying a lot, and I felt something was wrong. We went back to the doctor, and I told him I thought something was wrong. I wanted him to take off the cast and check things out. He really did not want to do that as he was afraid it was too early and would affect the outcome. I deferred to his judgment, and we returned home.

Cindy's irritability continued, and I was becoming more upset by it. She was crying often and not sleeping well. It was not like her. We returned to the doctor, and I insisted he remove the cast and check it. I had now developed an assertiveness I never had before. When he took the cast off, he found the pins in her knee were so long that when the cast dried it was putting pressure on the pins and moving them. It was definitely painful for her. He trimmed the pins and recast her leg and she returned to her usual good temperament. From that experience, that doctor learned to pay more attention to his patient's reactions and what I considered communication, as well as to have more respect for parental input.

Several months later, her foot was amputated. Before that surgery, a resident came in to talk with us and have us sign some papers. At one point in the process, he paused and seemed uncomfortable about the next form.

"What do you want to do with the foot?" he asked abruptly.

"You can release it to a funeral director but that would be costly and, in my opinion, silly. Or you can donate it for research and maybe help someone else."

I was so taken aback by his tone of voice and his lack of compassion that I was speechless. We were not talking about a piece of furniture but a part of our daughter. Even though the foot was of no use to her, it was still a part of her and it was difficult to give permission to have it cut off. Making that kind of life-changing decision was very difficult. But we had to make the decision just as we would have to continue to do for the rest of her life. It has never gotten easier, nor have we ever taken it lightly. Of course, we did not have the amputated foot released to a funeral director, but we did have our own private way of saying goodbye and we told Cindy we loved her just as much with or without it.

Once again, Cindy came through the surgery with flying colors. She came out of the surgery with a cast that had an artificial foot attached and a drainage tube sticking out from it. Right after the surgery, Cindy seemed to be in distress again. She was crying a lot, so much that she became nasal. When I asked to see a doctor, one of the residents looked at her briefly, said she had an upper respiratory infection, and had her put into a misting tent. I told them I thought they were wrong and that she was stuffed up because she was crying so hard, not because she had an infection. They scolded me for removing her from the misting tent to hold her even though I continued to tell them that was not the problem. She was crying very hard, and I was trying to comfort her. They refused to do anything else for her or listen to me, so I got on the phone and called her surgeon's office and demanded to see him.

A little later her doctor came to the ward, and I told him that Cindy was not acting right and I felt something was wrong someplace. I told the doctor I didn't think the tent was necessary because the problem was elsewhere. I told him that Cindy was telling us that something somewhere was wrong. He looked at me for a moment.

"You think something is wrong like when the pins were wrong?" he asked. I said yes it was the same thing. He pulled the drainage tube from her cast.

"Let's see if that does the trick." It did, she settled down, and shortly after the tent was removed. Cindy had taught him well.

OUR BIGGEST REGRET

The surgery on Cindy's leg proved to be much more complicated and difficult than we had thought. I do not know whether we really didn't understand what we were told or if we were intentionally misled. I think it was more the latter, but it may have been both. The initial surgery only positioned her lower limb, so an additional surgery was needed as it was still considerably bent. Once again, after the surgery she had a cast. But what followed was what I can only describe as torture. Every two weeks for eight weeks, her leg would be recast, and while it was wet, the doctor would stretch her leg and hold it until the cast dried. Cindy would cry for days, and two weeks later the process would be repeated. Neither Bob nor I remember being told about this part. I cannot believe we would have agreed to it. All the pain she endured was in hope of the possibility of her having only an artificial foot. Tragically, that never happened.

Cindy spent most of the first two years of her life in and out of the hospital. By the age of twelve, she underwent fourteen operations. Most of them were in the first few years of her life. But of all of them, the orthopedic surgeries and what followed, have had the most impact on her. She endured tremendous pain.

Bob and I have often talked, and we both agree that if each of us could change one and only one decision in our entire lives, it would be the decision we made regarding her leg. Even though it was an informed one, and we thought at the time it was the right one, we know now it was not. We had said at the time that we would explain our choice to Cindy someday not knowing at the time that it would not be possible. It is hard for us, and I still feel guilty about it. I wish I could talk to her about it and tell her how sorry I am but I cannot. We promised ourselves at the time we would not beat up on ourselves if it was the wrong decision, because we were told we had a 50/50 chance it would be successful. We did what we thought was the best thing for Cindy. But of course, it was not the right decision and ended up being the cause of many other problems.

Many years later, when we had Cindy's amputation revised to an above-the-knee one, the man who made her prosthesis made a comment to me.

"It never really stood much of a chance of working."

"That's not what we were told," I said in shock. He just looked at me and said no more.

Thinking back now, I wonder just how much of what that doctor told us was truthful. Were we purposely misled or not told of the extent of the surgeries and what would follow? Was he looking for someone to experiment on with this procedure? This was a teaching hospital after all. Despite our promise to each other, Bob and I both still feel guilt and anger about it. The doctor left the area shortly after Cindy's surgery, so I never was able to talk with him about it.

CINDY WILL SHOW HIM

The toll of all the surgeries caused Cindy to become fearful of doctors and hospitals, and she started to fight during procedures. One time while in the hospital, a doctor was trying to start an IV and Cindy was resisting. They insisted she have it as she was not eating well. When the doctor was finally successful, Cindy pulled it out. It was reinserted and she pulled it out again. I think they were surprised by Cindy's strength and determination.

Finally, the doctor decided he would insert a much longer and thinner line into her hand that would be more difficult to pull out. He had a very difficult time putting the line in partly because Cindy was fighting and crying so hard and he was sweating profusely. At one point he got up to take a break for a moment.

"How can you as her mother stand there and watch this?" he said in a condemning tone.

"I am here for my daughter no matter how difficult it is for me because it is not nearly as difficult as it is for her. If she can take it, so can I." He said no more.

When he was done, he strapped her hand to a board to immobilize it and then loosely tied her hands to the crib so she could still slightly move her arms but couldn't reach the tube to pull it.

"There is no way she will pull that one out," he said defiantly.

"Don't ever underestimate my daughter," I replied. "She has a mind of her own."

Cindy could barely move her hand as it was heavily taped but she would flex her fingers just a little and ever so slightly move her hand up and down. It took her a while but eventually she got it out. They could not believe it but I could, because Cindy was a fighter and not one to give up on what she wanted. I marveled at her perseverance and strength and I was inspired by it. The doctor finally gave up on the IV. I pleaded with her surgeon to let me take Cindy home where I thought she would do much better and would start eating. He agreed with me. Once she was home, Cindy started eating and quickly improved.

THERE WERE HAPPY TIMES TOO

Despite all the medical issues we were dealing with, there were also many happy times. We quietly celebrated each small advance Cindy made and enjoyed all the wonders of infancy that most parents do. No, the usual milestones were not there, but we probably appreciated the little things more than anyone.

During that first year, when we were between surgeries, I even managed to take a vacation. My parents had returned to Florida, and Cindy and I flew down and spent some time with them. It was a time when they could be grandparents and show off their new grandchild, and they did just that. They had a professional photographer take pictures of her, and one hung on their wall until the day they died. It is now one of Cindy's favorite pictures and is in her home.

On her first birthday we had a party. It was a milestone that few people thought she would reach, and we made a big deal of it. It helped to make up for the celebration we never got to have when she was born. We still had much to deal with but we were so proud and happy and grateful we had gotten as far as we did. Cindy surprised us all and especially her doctors. Despite all she had been through, she was incredibly good natured when not in the hospital. She was a good baby and smiled a great deal. She was truly a joy.

Chapter 2
MAKING AN IMPACT

My childhood was not what I would describe as a happy one. My parents were good people but not a good match. They had a difficult marriage and fought all the time. As a small child, I would sit at the top of the stairs and listen to them argue. I was convinced the only reason they were together was because of my brother and me and not because of any love between them. It was a relationship with no affection and constant bickering. My father was a well-known artist who enjoyed his work tremendously and was well-liked and respected in the community. He was very social and was often invited to community events, which he loved attending. My mother did not enjoy the social outings at all and only went to functions that she absolutely could not get out of. While my mother had a sharp business and political mind, socially she had serious issues. I was much more like my dad, and when I was young, he began to take me to many of the social functions. My teenage years were miserable for me, and I constantly fought with my mother. I was never able to please her or win her approval. She never trusted me or respected me, and she questioned my every move.

I had very little self-esteem when I was in high school. Like most teenagers, I wanted to be popular and be accepted into the in-crowd. But I was not, and there were only a few dates with guys from school. Most of my dates were a result of my brother, who was conveniently three years older and would often introduce me to his friends, including my husband. I was certainly not assertive and had great difficulty standing before my peers in class. Even in junior high school, I could not speak in front of the class without shaking so badly that many were laughing at me.

In my senior year of high school, as a requirement of English class, I had to give a five-minute talk. This terrified me, so both my parents helped me with it. My topic was optical illusions, and my dad, a professional artist, created magnificent charts illustrating them. I practiced my speech for weeks until I had it down perfectly. It was to be no less than four minutes and no more than six. I was consistently at five minutes. I was sure I could do it. I got so nervous when I stood in front of the class that my notecards fell to the floor, the charts went flying off the easel, and my five-minute speech was barely two minutes. My classmates were laughing, and I was on the verge of tears. Standing in front of the class was just not my cup of tea.

I was never able to talk with my mother or confide in her. I truly felt she neither liked nor loved me. I was miserable and had few things in life that gave me pleasure. I did enjoy singing and was part of the school chorus. I even got a small singing part in the school play. I was incredibly proud and excited, but my mother had some excuse to not come see it. I was not happy in high school and was glad to see it end. I am not sure my mother even came to my graduation. If she did, I am sure she let me know how awful it was for her and how much she did not want to go. Our relationship was a difficult and confrontational one and continued that way even after I went away to college.

I could not wait to go to college as it meant I could get away from home and that is what I wanted most. For some strange reason, I thought I wanted to be a teacher and went to the State University of New York at Oswego to pursue that. I am not sure that is what I wanted, but it was as good a choice as anything. I must have been insane at the time to even consider a career where I would be standing in front of a class all day. What was I thinking? But Oswego was about forty miles away, an hour drive from home, and I would live on campus.

Wouldn't you know it with my luck one of the required courses my freshman year was public speaking. When I found out about that, I almost quit school before I even started. I needed to take it either first or second semester and decided to get it over with as soon as possible. I figured it was a sure F.

I had a great teacher and I paid close attention. Toward the end of the semester, as I feared, I was required to give a speech to the class. Two things we had been taught really stuck in my mind. They were to talk about something you really know and to try to get the audience's attention early.

"Do you know that there is a parade on campus every Friday afternoon?" I began.

The very puzzled looks from my fellow students told me I had their attention. I then explained that the parade was the stream of students going to Bucklands, the local bar in town, and that was the topic of my talk. It was something I knew well and the class could certainly relate to it.

Shortly after my speech, the teacher asked to see me in her office. I thought for sure she was going to chew me out for my choice of topics. Instead, she asked me if I would be interested in joining the debate team. I think I burst out laughing and told her no way. I could not possibly do that. She told me she thought I would be great and asked me to think about it. I sure was not ready to be a part of that team, but the lessons she taught in that class proved to be useful and right on target in the not-too-distant future. And, I got an A minus on that talk and a course grade of a B. Ironically, it was to be the best performance in my college career.

I did not do well in school and never finished. I had too much fun at Bucklands, where I spent far too much time. I worked harder on my social life than on my courses, and eventually it caught up with me. Unfortunately, leaving school meant moving back home. I was going to night school for a while but when I took a job with an airline, night school was history. The choice between traveling and studying did not require too much thought on my part. I still wanted to have a good time.

Even after I was earning my own money and doing well in my job with the airline, my relationship with my mother continued to be strained and difficult. I still felt she would criticize or question my every move. She would often drink heavily, and when she did, she became mean. There were times she embarrassed me in public. I lived at home for a while but moved into an apartment with a friend as soon as financially possible, once again, so I could get away from home.

CINDY MENDS A RELATIONSHIP

It was not until I married, became pregnant, and started having problems that my relationship with my mother changed dramatically. She seemed to have a new respect for me. When Cindy was born, she and my father were, of course, devastated by all her problems. But they both adored her, and in their eyes, Cindy was an angel who could do no wrong. My mother especially had a special connection with Cindy. For some unknown reason, my mother had a terrible fear of choking to death, so Cindy's difficulties with eating really hit home with her. She greatly admired her and the way she dealt with all the feeding issues, and Cindy won her over on that alone.

Ironically, years later my mother would develop COPD, congestive heart failure, and was diagnosed with ALS, or Lou Gehrig's disease. She would lose her ability to swallow properly, and speech was difficult. Choking became a real possibility for her. She told me several times that watching Cindy struggle with the feeding issues as a baby helped her deal with all she was going through. She often told me how much she admired and respected Cindy for the way she had handled all her medical issues. Fortunately, my mother died peacefully in her sleep.

Even though my parents lived far away when Cindy was born, they were still a great source of comfort to me. There were many lengthy long-distance calls and letters. My mother and I had a new relationship, and we became quite close. Cindy had brought us together. I shared my emotions with her and learned I could confide in her. She obviously had a new respect for both Bob and me and frequently told us how much she loved and admired us. She had definitely softened; she still had her own issues, but we became more understanding and tolerant of them. Except for Bob and me, my mother loved Cindy the most of anyone and always accepted her as she was from day one. She never showed one ounce of embarrassment or shame but only incredible pride and admiration. And if ever anyone did not show Cindy proper respect, she would get furious. When it came to Cindy, any shyness or lack of confidence my mother had in the past went right out the window, and she was one of Cindy's strongest advocates.

CINDY TEACHES ME TO BE ASSERTIVE

Cindy returned to the hospital many times during the first two years of her life. Although she was progressing nicely feeding on her own, the gastrostomy tube remained. We had regular appointments with Dr. Franco for check-ups, and there were several emergency room visits. One time I called in a panic because I thought she had something caught in her throat. He saw her immediately, and it turned out she was just fine. I apologized over and over. Dr. Franco smiled and told me there was no need to apologize and I should not hesitate to call him anytime I felt there was something wrong. He was such a wonderful, caring, and compassionate man. Although she was fine that time, Cindy did have to have her esophagus dilated again but in spite continued to progress with eating normally.

We relied less and less on the feeding tube, and at one point, Cindy even pulled the tube out when she was in the hospital for another procedure. We felt she was telling us she didn't need it or want it anymore. The doctor wanted to put it back, and she was scheduled for another surgery to do that. When the papers giving permission were presented to me, I did not want to sign them. I told the resident I wanted to speak with Dr. Franco himself because I didn't feel she needed the tube any longer. The resident told me Dr. Franco was in surgery and I had to sign the papers. I refused to do so until I could speak directly to the doctor and hear his reasons for wanting to put it back in.

Once again, I was the talk of the floor and was now quickly becoming a nuisance to them. Sometimes when I got to the hospital, I would feel like the staff were saying, "Oh boy, here she comes." I was learning to question everything and not take anything for granted. I expected to be treated with respect and for Cindy to be also. It would be a lesson I would learn again and again. Dr. Franco came to see me between surgeries, and we discussed his reasons for wanting to put the tube back in. We had a mutual respect, and he was not at all put out by my wanting to speak to him first. Of course, I deferred to his judgment and signed the papers. Later it proved to be the right thing to do. I was learning how to work with professionals and have a mutual respectful relationship even when it was incredibly difficult. And I no longer had a problem speaking up or being assertive. Cindy changed all that.

CINDY INSTILLS CONFIDENCE IN ME

From the day Cindy was born, I was in awe of her. I watched her struggle and fight and I drew strength from her. Because of her I learned to do things I would not have thought I could do. I became more confident in myself and my abilities because of her. I learned to believe in myself and trust my instincts. Cindy opened a whole new world for me and one in which I learned a great deal. I developed a passion or mission, if you will, because of her.

Over the years I even overcame my fears of public speaking. After I left the workforce, I would return years later on a part-time basis teaching classes about parents' rights under the education law. I became a teacher after all, and enjoyed it immensely. I spoke at conferences and presented testimony at various forums. I became an advocate for people with disabilities. All these changes and new abilities were because of Cindy. She has made my life better in so many ways. Because of Cindy I think I am a better person.

Chapter 3
PROBLEMS, QUESTIONS, AND DISCOVERIES

All through the first three years, we had endless appointments, including the heart specialist. Cindy had several cardiac problems, but they turned out not to be as severe as they first thought. She had dextrocardia, which means her heart is turned around or, as some describe it, on the wrong side. This by itself does not pose a problem if the heart is functioning properly. She also had a ventricular septal defect (VSD), or a hole in the wall between the two chambers, as well as pulmonary stenosis, a thickening of the pulmonary artery. These could cause some problems and would be monitored closely. Fortunately, she did not have the fourth defect they originally suspected at birth.

The appointments with the pediatric cardiac specialist were an awful ordeal. Every one was scheduled at noon, and when you arrived, the waiting room was filled beyond capacity. Because patients were seen on a first-come basis, I usually tried to get there early so I could be higher on the sign-in list and at least get a seat in the waiting room. We would wait for hours before being called to have an EKG. I would undress Cindy, who would usually cry and fuss and struggle. In those days the machines were not as sophisticated as they are now, and Cindy had to stay perfectly still for quite a while, which was a real challenge. After that, I would dress her again and return to the waiting area where we would wait for the next step. Once again, we would be called and put in a room where I would undress her one more time for an exam. We would wait in the exam room until a doctor came and did the exam. Then I would dress her and return to the waiting room again to wait to speak with the doctor. Finally, we would be called to his office to hear the results.

The appointments were an all-day ordeal, and by the time I got home, I felt like I was the one who needed a heart doctor. Considering everything, I thought Cindy did incredibly well, probably better than me. Her first cardiologist was an older man who was very stern and would yell at me if my eyes were not directed at the model he was using or if I was not reacting the way he thought I should. He was clinically an excellent doctor but not a people person. He retired after a few years and was replaced by an excellent female doctor, Dr. White, who had a wonderful and compassionate nature. The appointments weren't any shorter as they were still booked the same way, but I had great respect for Dr. White.

We were fortunate that over the years the hole between the chambers of Cindy's heart healed itself over, and the pulmonary stenosis proved not to be a problem, so no surgery was required. I always felt that Cindy's heart must have been pretty strong in order to endure all that she did. She is now regularly monitored by her internist as well as periodically with a cardiologist, and antibiotics are given before certain procedures.

DEALING WITH THE ANGER

I have heard that when a child with a disability is born, the parents go through the same five stages of grief experienced with a death. That is easy to understand because you experience the death of the healthy, normal child you dreamed about. I went through those stages vacillating from one to another. There were many angry stages and those were sometimes very difficult to get through, so I sought professional help along the way. Sometimes that anger got in the way and interfered with my ability to communicate. Specifically, I was angry at Dr. Schaffer for the way he had delivered the news about Cindy when she was born. And I was especially angry about the way he told me of the need to amputate her leg. This anger was so intense that I started avoiding him. I finally decided to deal with it. At the appropriate time and place, I asked for some time to talk with him.

"I want you to know I have a problem with the manner in which you told us about our daughter when she was born, as well as the news about her leg," I said calmly. His response surprised me.

"I don't think there was any way I could have delivered that kind of news so that you would have taken it well, but I admit that my way may not have been the best." He went on with a sympathetic and an apologetic tone.

"These things are difficult for doctors too, and we learn from our experiences, and I have learned from yours."

I thought about what he said, and his words hit home. Was I angry at him or the circumstances? Was it the messenger or the message? No, he probably did not do it in the most sensitive way, but I realized it was more than his method that was causing my anger. When I left his office that day, I felt a weight had been lifted from me. I had dealt with a piece of anger I had never let go of before. And I recognized I needed to deal with the rest of it.

It also helped to meet other parents who shared and understood some of our experiences. I became involved with a parent group early on that was associated with our local Cerebral Palsy Center. Cindy went there for her therapies and clinical evaluations. Our group met often and shared a great deal about our children and our lives in general. The group was led by a fellow parent who was also a psychologist. We laughed and cried together and felt so comfortable with one another that there was very little we could not say in front of each other. We all learned from one another and our experiences. Although the group has not met in many years, some of us remain friends and continue to see each other. That kind of support and camaraderie is lifelong, and these are people I still feel I can say anything to about my child. They will understand.

WHY DID THIS HAPPEN?

One of the questions that came up in my mind often is, of course, "Why me?" Some parents had an answer to that because their child's disability was the result of medical malpractice or a birth injury or even an inherited or acquired disease. But we did not have a reason, and my initial fears when I first became pregnant still haunted me. Bob's mom told me shortly after Cindy's birth that there was "none of that in our family." As soon as I suspected I was pregnant, I know I acted responsibly. I did not drink, have never smoked, and did not take any kind of drugs or even over-the-counter medicines. But the question of whether I had something to do with all this still nagged at me. I even asked the pediatrician one day if my love of tanning myself on the beach could have caused any of Cindy's problems. He assured me that although there were many things they did not know about the causes of such defects, it was definitely not from lying in the sun. He did suggest that we think about consulting a geneticist.

When Cindy was just over a year old, we were referred to a well-known and highly respected doctor specializing in genetics who had many world-recognized publications. During the evaluation, Cindy had blood tests and we answered many questions. When we met with the doctor and his resident to hear the results of his evaluation, they told us that the blood tests showed all Cindy's chromosomes were normal. Therefore, this was not genetic, and there was no reason we should not have more children.

"It won't happen again." That was, of course, good news to us but what followed was not. Because Cindy's chromosomes were all normal, there was no clear-cut syndrome in which to classify her such as Down Syndrome, a mutation of a specific chromosome. So, their finding was a clinical diagnosis based on her combination of defects and facial features, such as the shape of her nose. They told us she had Cornelia DeLange Syndrome. Of course, we had no idea what that was or what it meant. They spoke in some terms that meant nothing to us or with which we had little experience. We were told she would have at best an IQ of 15 or 20. I remember we both were so overwhelmed with it all that we asked how high an IQ one needed to graduate from high school. The response was that one would probably need an IQ of 90 or so. We were told we should expect very little of Cindy and that she probably would not progress much more than the point she was at right then. They were pretty much telling us she would be a vegetable.

I do not think we totally realized the impact of what we were being told at the time or maybe we were just too shocked to be able to think clearly, but once again we were devastated. All our hopes and dreams for our child had been shattered. When we returned home and started talking, once again, we held each other and cried. I think this was the second and last time I wondered if her surviving all she had was indeed the best thing.

I do not think that we ever totally accepted what was said to us that day. After all, we knew Cindy so well and had watched her come so far it was hard to believe what they told us. So, after the initial shock and grief, I think we put it aside and chose to ignore it. Unfortunately, others did not do the same. What we did not realize was that the diagnosis would follow Cindy and have a tremendous impact on her life.

CAN CINDY HEAR?

Cindy was receiving lots of therapies but some of the people working with her just did not seem to have their heart in it. They were very pessimistic about her prognosis, and when I would ask what I could do to help her, they would say "nothing" or just shrug. Many of the people working with Cindy showed little interest or enthusiasm in what they were doing.

Cindy was also getting many ear infections. Her ear, nose, and throat (ENT) specialist decided she needed tubes in her ears, which required another trip to the OR. During one of the follow-up appointments with the ENT specialist, I questioned whether Cindy could hear. I will never forget his stern response as he looked me straight in the eyes.

"Now Mrs. Kantak, I am your doctor, listen to me. You have to accept it, your daughter is not deaf, she is hopelessly retarded."

Once more, the professionals were telling me one thing and my instincts were telling me something different. Cindy was able to sleep through anything. We lived close to a ballpark and on a hot summer night when the windows were open, the fireworks never woke her up. Because she still required feeding during the night, I would easily go into her room without ever waking her and give her formula through the G tube. No matter how much noise I made, she would not wake up until the formula went through the tube into her stomach.

At about the same time, my brother suggested I meet with a friend of his, Mark, who was a pediatrician and worked for the New York State Office of Mental Retardation and Developmental Disability (OMRDD). I had not hooked up with this agency yet so I thought it was a good idea. On my first visit with Mark, I expressed my concern about the hearing and the doctor's comment. His reaction was to find out for sure one way or another. So he referred us to the Communications Disorder Unit (CDU) associated with a local hospital.

Although Cindy was uncooperative and difficult to test, they found she did indeed have a hearing loss although they were not able to ascertain the extent of the loss. They did, however, feel it was significant and recommended hearing aids. It was another blow for us, more bad news, but worse, it was a huge loss for Cindy. She was almost three years old and had lost all that precious time. I remembered back when she was just an infant in the hospital just before she came home the second time, I questioned her hearing back then. The resident I spoke with was the same one I had had words with before over the tube in her nose. He banged his little hammer against the crib several times and Cindy startled. He then said she could hear. I was still somewhat naïve back then. It was a metal crib and the vibration and the movement of the crib are what woke her. Boy, if I had known then what I know now, her hearing loss would have been discovered much sooner. Another huge regret and source of guilt for me. If only I had persisted.

After discovering her hearing loss, it became quite clear to me why we were having trouble getting people to work with Cindy and why they were so pessimistic. The prognosis given to her by the geneticist was so bleak that people thought no matter how hard they worked, there would be no progress. Of course, Cindy's lack of response was viewed as part of that hopelessness and not of the fact she could not hear.

At Mark's suggestion, we returned to the geneticist for re-evaluation. After seeing Cindy again and learning of her deafness, he told us he had made a terrible mistake. Her facial features and the handicaps no longer fit into the previously diagnosed syndrome. Now he had a new name or label for her. This time it was called VATER syndrome. When we asked what the potential IQ would be with this one, we were told it could be as high as borderline to low average.

"Do you have any idea how much of an impact this mistake has had on our daughter's life?" I screamed at him.

"For well over a year, we have had people refuse to work with her or not listen to our concerns because of your prognosis." My voice was filled with anger. I completely lost control.

He gave us what I suppose was an apology, but it was not enough. To his credit, he sat and took my outburst offering no excuses. When his assistant walked me out, he turned to me and said he did not blame me one bit for my anger and that he would have done the same thing. While I appreciated his empathy, it did not negate what had happened. The doctor's incorrect label caused Cindy to lose crucial and precious time that could never be regained. The loss of that time and its repercussions would have a lifelong impact.

I insisted that the doctor rewrite his report and see that everyone who had received the prior report remove it from her file. I have no way of knowing if that was done, but there has never been any mention of the first diagnosis. After this new report went out, people seemed to change their attitudes toward Cindy for the better, and they were more enthusiastic in their work.

SOMETIMES IT IS WHO YOU KNOW

We were also referred to a program run by our county called the Physically Handicapped Children's Program, which would help with some of the many medical expenses. Although Bob had very good insurance coverage through his employer, they did not cover everything. We went through the application process, giving them complete financial and social histories. It would be the first of many times I would do that. In fact, we would have to do it so many times in so many different situations that I would often tease about it. I told people I was tempted to run a full-page ad in the newspaper entitled "Everything you want to know about the Kantak family. Now please do not ask me again." Privacy no longer existed for us. Our life was an open book.

Now that we knew Cindy was deaf, we wanted to get her hearing aids as quickly as possible. She had already lost three years of a critical time for learning. We were told the approval for the hearing aids may take as long as six months to come through, and they could not be ordered until it did. I was furious and pleaded for them to make an exception but was unsuccessful in convincing them. I could not believe under the circumstances they were going to make us wait even longer. Bob happened to bowl in a league with someone who had a brother involved in local politics. He had casually mentioned the problem we were having, and this friend mentioned it to his brother. A few days later, we were told to contact an aide in the office of one of our state senators. I relayed my story to him, and he said he would see what he could do. In less than a week, we had our approval. It was my first lesson in the power of political connections and how you sometimes need to circumvent the system.

The Communications Disorder Unit (CDU) continued to test Cindy on a regular basis. Cindy was enrolled in the early developmental program operated by the local Cerebral Palsy Center, where she had her program a couple of days a week and all her therapies. Because of the continual difficulty in testing Cindy over the years, when she was five years old, the CDU recommended she go to Rochester, New York, about ninety miles away, for a BSER or brainstem evoked response test. This test could more accurately determine the extent of Cindy's hearing loss. During this test, she was sedated and electrodes were put on her head much the same as an EEG to measure if the nerves are conducting the sound. It was not a painful or invasive procedure but it was yet another procedure for Cindy to endure, and she was not happy about it. We had to give her the maximum amount of medicine to get her to sleep. The test confirmed that she had a severe to profound hearing loss in both ears.

EATING PROBLEMS

Although Cindy's progress was truly remarkable, she still had many problems. Eating was always difficult as her esophagus just did not function as it should. When she first began eating solid food, she had difficulty handling it and would throw up at almost every meal. If she put too much food in her mouth or we gave her the wrong food, it just would not go down because of the inability of the esophagus to expand normally due to the scar tissue. It made mealtime very difficult for us, but she had to learn to handle the food. Of course, we were very careful about what we gave her, and eventually she learned how to eat, but for many years, dinner was not a pleasant time.

Even today, she still has problems with certain foods, and there are some things she needs to stay away from or be careful of. For instance, many years ago she ate a yellow marshmallow chick, the kind that is popular around Easter. It had been sitting around for a day and was slightly stale and no longer soft. We received a call from her housemate saying that Cindy seemed to be in distress and had her head bowed as if she was having trouble swallowing it. I made sure she was not having trouble breathing and was not choking and advised those with her I would be right there and if she got any worse to call an ambulance. By the time I got to her, she had drunk enough water to melt and dissolve it and was all right.

Another time, her housemate thought she had the flu because she was vomiting. She kept her in bed and gave her liquids. A day or so later, when she appeared to be better, she took her out to breakfast for pancakes. Although she was in good spirits and eager to eat, she got sick again. I was called, and they came right over to our house. After observing her, we knew that something was stuck in her throat and she needed to go to the hospital. We contacted her doctor and took her to the emergency room.

After an exam, she was sent for a barium swallow. Cindy was very nervous but cooperative nonetheless. I acted as an interpreter for the technician, signing his instructions. When she began to drink the liquid, he immediately had me stop her. I also watched the test on the screen and saw how her esophagus handled the thick liquid. First, it was obvious that there was some kind of blockage and very little was getting through. But what really struck me was seeing her esophagus and the scar tissue's effect on it. The normal part of it expanded a great deal but the repaired part remained so incredibly small. I had always understood the problem and condition, but seeing it like that gave me a new respect and awe for what Cindy had accomplished. The test showed there was something there that needed to be removed. Normally, they would do the procedure right in the ER, but because of her disabilities, it was determined she would have to be scheduled for the OR the next day.

We had learned a long time before this that we could not leave Cindy alone in the hospital, and this time proved no different. Cindy was in a room with a huge sign over her bed "NPO," which means nothing by mouth. Around dinner time, a nurse or an aide brought in a tray of food and set it in front of Cindy.

"Why are you bringing her that?" I asked while pointing to the sign.

"That is only after midnight, the standard for pre-op patients," she responded.

"Take that away and check her chart," I demanded. "She has a blockage."

She put the tray on the table near the next bed and sighed as she left the room. In a few minutes, she came back in and took the tray away and never said a word. It was incidents like this that were the reason we would not leave Cindy alone. Her inability to communicate posed too many problems. Bob and I took shifts around the clock, so one of us was always with her. I even went into the OR holding area as well as the OR post-op area so that I could sign to her and be with her. It was something I became used to doing, and usually the nurses welcomed my help.

As it turned out Cindy had what appeared to be a piece of steak caught in her throat. The doctor removed it and dilated her esophagus while she was there. When I asked her housemate, I found out that she had hosted a barbecue a few days earlier. Although someone had been careful to cut away the gristle on the steak, they did not remove it from the plate and Cindy ate it all.

When Cindy attended a day care center, she required another emergency trip to the hospital. She still had some difficulty eating, and everyone who worked with her was cautioned about the foods she could not have. Unfortunately, one day one of the other kids fed Cindy some kind of trail mix that included peanuts, and it stuck in her throat. She was not having trouble breathing so you wouldn't know until she tried to eat and nothing would go down. During another trip to the OR, the blockage was removed and her esophagus dilated once more.

CINDY'S FEARS

In the early years, one of the most difficult aspects of everything Cindy had been through was that she became so afraid of everything. Whenever we got in the car and got on the main highway that went through the city, Cindy would start screaming. She equated that road with going to the hospital. She also had difficulty going any place that she was unfamiliar with, even a grocery store. If she knew where she was going and she was secure about that, she was just fine but if she didn't then she screamed loud and long. This was understandable although it made things very difficult for us.

The impact of all she had been through really hit home with us one time when Cindy started screaming during her programs and therapies at the Cerebral Palsy Center (CP Center). We could not understand it because she had been going there for some time and had been just fine.

We had a meeting with everyone involved to brainstorm what could be done. During the meeting, I suddenly realized that we had just returned from a trip to Florida to see my parents. Twice before I had taken a trip and both times when we had returned Cindy went into the hospital for surgery. She had remembered that and was feeling scared and must have thought she was going to have surgery again. A behavior modification program was implemented immediately where her therapists and teacher held her and comforted her when she began screaming. Soon she settled down and felt secure once again. She was teaching us how smart she was and what a memory she had and that we needed to pay attention to that. Once we had the ability to communicate with her in sign language, it became somewhat easier because we could tell her where we were going.

Cindy still had problems going any place not familiar to her and would cry when she did. It made taking her places extremely difficult and nerve-racking, so one summer Bob and I along with my parents decided to try to change that. My parents would put Cindy in the car and sit in the driveway. While she screamed, they would hold her close and comfort her, never leaving the driveway. Then when she was accustomed to that, they would drive her around the block, comfort her while she screamed, and bring her back. When she became comfortable with that, they would go a little farther. They did this for weeks.

Bob and I would take her to the grocery store or get on the route that always frightened her and constantly reassure her that she was safe. We took many rides in the car in order to decondition her and make her understand that these places did not necessarily mean the hospital or doctor. Once a week while Bob was golfing, I picked Cindy up from daycare and took her to a restaurant, something else we could not do without her screaming. Each week I would take her to a place and tell them when I went in that I might not stay long, and they would have to bring me the check quickly if I needed to go. I got some very strange looks. I had to leave quickly many times. I never went to the same restaurant more than once, but over the period of a couple of months, I was finally able to take Cindy to a restaurant and order and eat an entire meal. Today, eating out is one of her favorite things to do.

Sometimes when Cindy would scream, we thought it was out of fear but we were wrong. Once when she and I flew to Florida to visit my parents, I had a prescribed sedative to give her if she was upset on the plane. I gave her the prescribed dose before the flight and hoped for the best. Unfortunately, it did not help, and Cindy started screaming during the flight. I gave her another dose up to the allowed maximum, but it just did not work. Nothing I did would calm her down and I was feeling uncomfortable. There were some very ignorant people sitting in front of us who were downright rude. They kept making awful remarks about us and complaining to the flight attendant, saying things like they did not understand why I let the kid get away with it. They would spank her for sure. They demanded a seat change, which was not possible, and even demanded we be removed from the plane immediately. It was a nonstop flight. Even the stewardess was annoyed with them and asked if she could do anything for me and told me to try not to let them upset me. I told her that hitting her certainly wouldn't help and I was doing everything I could but I thought she was scared.

   A lovely lady across the aisle was observing this and came over to me and struck up a conversation. She was very nice and offered to sit with Cindy if I wanted to go wash my face or just take a walk up the aisle. When we finally got off the plane, my father met us; I could not wait to get out of there. While waiting for our baggage, my father ran into someone he knew who was on the same plane. I told him I was the one with the screaming kid, and he assured me that many others had been there too. I had attributed her screaming to her fear of strange places. What I did not know until a day later, when she started running a fever, is that she had an ear infection. She was given an antibiotic and on the flight back a week later, she was just fine with no sedation. In fact, she was smiling the entire trip and never missed anything going on. Today, flying is another of Cindy's favorite things to do. She loves to travel.

A SIXTH SENSE?

I have always felt that because Cindy is deaf, her other senses are heightened. She has always had an ability to sense how someone feels about her. If they are afraid of her for any reason, she will know it and probably take advantage of that. If someone is intimidated by her, she will be intimidating. She also knows when someone feels warmth and affection for her and will respond the same way. She has always been able to notice our moods even when we are careful about not showing them. When Bob's brother was ill with cancer, Cindy sat on the side of his bed and just smiled at him. I am sure she knew he was in pain and felt a special bond with him.

One summer while attending a day camp, Cindy rode to the camp on a bus hired out to a private company. We never hid her artificial leg or hearing aids, and when the weather permitted, she always wore shorts. At the beginning of one summer, she would board the bus each morning, and the driver would stare at her, particularly at her leg. It was not a look of concern making sure she boarded OK but one almost of revulsion. I had become used to people staring so I ignored it, but Cindy would stop momentarily and look back at him.

Toward the end of the first week, when he continued to do it, Cindy stopped and grabbed his arm. It startled him, he looked her in the eye, and she just stared at him. Her look was worth a thousand words, and it was much more effective than anything I could have said to the man. He never stared at her like that again. She taught him a valuable lesson I hope has remained with him.

Cindy understands time as it related to things in her life. She senses when a holiday is approaching, perhaps by the weather or other indicators. She knows there is an order to holidays. Almost as soon as we finished our Thanksgiving dinner, she would want the Christmas decorations pulled out. The approach of warmer weather meant the end of school and the start of summer activities. While specific days and months on the calendar may not have been totally understood, she definitely could mark off days by the number of sleeps. To this day, we mark events on a calendar. Vacations are pointed out, and she is told how many sleeps.

In addition to her incredible memory, she also has a strong sense of direction. If we told her we were going to a certain place and we drove in a direction she was not used to when going there, she would actually point in the direction she wanted to go. There were some places we could almost have her direct us by pointing. One day when I was following our usual routine of taking her to daycare on my way to work, I was daydreaming and started driving directly to my office. Cindy tapped me on the arm and pointed back where I missed the turn. I nodded yes and thanked her, and we both laughed. For someone who was supposed to be a vegetable, she sure didn't miss a trick.

Cindy also possesses a distinct sense of order. As a child, her items had a place and order to them. A comb in the bathroom had to be in a certain place with the teeth facing a certain direction. Her stuffed animals were positioned a certain way. Unfortunately, as she grew older, this turned into an obsessive-compulsive disorder and poses some difficulties for her. Although she takes medication for this, there are times when it creeps in, especially when she is tired. She may stand and sit several times before completing the task. Or she may cross a threshold two or three times before entering a room completely.

A MIND OF HER OWN

Cindy continued to remind us that she had a mind of her own. When she was four years old, her orthopedic surgeries were done for the time being, and she was wearing a full-leg prosthesis with a stiff knee. We were trying to teach her to walk and being told her only hope lay in using a walker. Her physical therapist kept pushing us to force the walker on her, but Cindy kept pushing it away. I was scolded for not doing the right thing for Cindy and was told I was hurting her by not encouraging the walker. I continued to stress that Cindy was indicating to us that she did not want the walker. The therapist kept telling us it was her only hope. At the time, we had moved into a new house that had a big bow window in the living room. Cindy would crawl to the window, reach for the large sill, and pull herself up so she could see out. Bob and I began a routine of holding her between us and letting her balance for a split second. Gradually, she would stand for longer periods of time. Eventually, she took her first step and after that there was no stopping her. She did not walk on her own until she was almost five years old but she never used that walker. She knew what she wanted and she was going to do it her own way and in her own time.

Cindy attended a day care center housed in a local church. It was a wonderful program with terrific staff and it provided her with much needed socialization. They were very accepting of her despite her difficulties. The other children loved her, and she had one or two that she saw occasionally outside of daycare. One day when I picked her up several of the other children came up to me and told me they were going to teach Cindy how to walk. I have no doubt they played a huge role in her eventually walking. Nor did I doubt that Cindy left a lasting impression on them as well.

Also at this day care center, she met a teaching assistant named Maggie. Maggie worked closely with Cindy and took a strong liking to her. As a result of their relationship and the experience of working with Cindy, Maggie decided to go back to school to become a teacher for the deaf. She currently is just that and although she lives in Arizona, she keeps in touch with us and visited Cindy in her home several years ago. Cindy had made a lasting impression that many others would benefit from.

Despite all the difficulties, Cindy was really a happy child. When she was not feeling threatened, she smiled all the time and was loving and affectionate. She and I had a routine before each school day where she would sit on my lap or next to me and we would hug. Special times I will always cherish. She adored family get-togethers. She loved parties of any kind and would often intensely watch other people. We took Cindy many places, stores, on picnics and various outings, and some wonderful vacations.

Cindy has a wonderful sense of humor and sometimes finds humor in other people's mishaps. Once, while she was sitting at the breakfast table and I was loading the dishwasher, I accidentally lost my balance and fell backward over the door. The glass in my hand went flying along with me. Although I did end up with a dislocated patella, I must admit I probably looked pretty silly and could not blame Cindy for initially laughing. But she quickly understood that I was hurt and became instantly somber and worried. She is so keen to other people's emotions.

Chapter 4
FORMAL EDUCATION BEGINS

Eventually, we all settled into our routine of periodic medical appointments and therapies, and I was even able to return to my work at the insurance company on a part-time basis. Cindy was in an infant education program at our local CP Center and was also getting her therapies there. Now that she was no longer in a medical crisis, it was time to get her some educational services. Everything up to this point had been medically oriented. We were referred to an educational consultant, Sharon, who worked for the state, and she guided me through this process. She turned out to be both a wonderful advocate and a great teacher. She taught me a lot about advocacy and how to work the system.

Finding programs was difficult. The Educational for All Handicapped Children Act (PL94-142), now called IDEA, was passed the previous year, 1975, but had not yet had an impact. We managed to get Cindy into a preschool program at the local ARC (Association for Retarded Citizens). Although the teacher was not a certified teacher for the deaf, she did use sign language and began teaching Cindy signs. One of the first signs she learned was "happy," and despite all she had been through, that is exactly what she was. She smiled all the time and she loved being in school. They were also teaching her the letters in her first name, and Cindy invented her name sign — a "C" done in an upward motion at the chest just like the sign for happy. It was the perfect sign for her, and she has used it ever since. They also worked on all the usual preschool things, including a highly structured toilet-training procedure, an area where we had previously had no success.

CINDY IMPACTS POLICY

Shortly after Cindy began in the program, the school district informed me that they may not be able to transport her. Their policy was to transport preschool students on a space-available-only basis. If they had a bus going to the school with school-aged children on it, and if there was room, then they would transport. But if they needed that seat to transport a school-aged student, then Cindy would be bumped. I was told they would begin transporting her, but because they used the small buses, I could expect her to be bumped very shortly. I was outraged at this and felt it terribly unfair. I would never know from day to day if she would have transportation. It could be taken away at any time. I tried to rectify this through the proper school district channels with no success. I also tried outside sources of transportation with no luck. Sharon gave me the name of one of our school board members who happened to have a daughter who was deaf. I called him and he suggested I write a letter to the school board and possibly contact the superintendent directly. I ended up calling the superintendent at his home. I told him who I was and why I was calling.

"I do not think this policy is fair," I pleaded. He was not very receptive, most likely irritated that I called him at home. The conversation continued but was going nowhere. I upped the ante.

"I think this policy is discriminatory and if I need to go to the newspaper, I will do just that," I said confidently knowing my father worked for the paper.

"How dare you threaten me," he yelled. "I am insulted by your suggestion that we are doing something wrong. I am sure our policy is not discriminatory. I will consult our attorney tomorrow and get back to you," he said defiantly.

Two days later he called me with a much milder tone in his voice and told me that he would be bringing this matter to the board for discussion. They would decide what should be done. I followed up by writing a letter to the school board telling them of my transportation problem and everything I had done to try and resolve it. The school board member I spoke with earlier let me know when the matter was to come up and how I could give my input at the meeting. He also said he would call some other parents.

I attended the school board meeting and found out that they did have a problem with their busing policy. Either they had to bus all preschoolers or no preschoolers but they could not do some and not others. They had a decision to make. They could vote to not bus any preschool children and be within their rights. If that happened, Cindy as well as others would lose their transportation completely.

At the appropriate time I asked to speak and told the school board of the difficulties I was having and how I needed this transportation to maintain my job. I can't remember all I said, but I do remember how very difficult it was for me and how incredibly nervous I was at the time. Shades of my high school difficulties speaking before groups were still there. This was so unlike anything I had ever done before and I could not believe I did it. I was speaking in front of all these strangers. Cindy had inspired me and given me new strength and purpose.

After I spoke, to my amazement three other women, whom I had never seen or talked to before, also spoke in support of passing a policy to bus all the preschoolers. I was absolutely blown away by them and, afterward in the hallway, I quietly thanked them and thought what a wonderful thing for them to do. These were parents that the school board member had called, and they understood because they also had children with disabilities. They came to support me even though it would not benefit them directly. It was a very powerful lesson in the strength of numbers. I vowed that someday, somehow, I would return that favor to another parent. I never forgot that promise and welcome any opportunity to help another parent. I have given many talks and submitted testimony in forums advocating for people with disabilities, always remembering how helpful those three parents were to me.

The school board made the right decision and adopted a policy to bus all preschool children with disabilities. As a result of Cindy, this change in policy would help many others like her.

THOSE NASTY LABELS AGAIN

Because of Cindy's problems, it was difficult to test her. The psychologist at the ARC thought we should consider consulting with someone with experience testing the deaf. So we were referred to a psychologist about an hour away who specialized in testing children with hearing losses. We drove to see her and spent a couple of hours with her and Cindy. She also found it difficult to get accurate tests but managed better than most. When she sent her report to us, it stated the results of the tests she was able to perform. Cindy was five years old at the time but was unable to complete the testing at the two-year-old level, the minimum for computing an IQ. The Diagnostic Impression stated, "Cindy is a retarded child whose potential cannot yet be firmly stated." It also read, "There is, at present, no clear basis for expecting her to develop an IQ of 50 but it is too early to be certain." Fortunately, we were paying her fee ourselves, so the report came directly to us and only us. I told her this kind of a comment could be very detrimental to Cindy and told her the story of the geneticist. I was afraid of the same thing happening again. She understood my concern but felt I needed to know her opinion. After she made that clear, she agreed to revise her report to exclude that one sentence. Of course, it was the revised report that I released to the school district and others.

In those days students with mental retardation were classified for educational purposes into two categories: educable mentally retarded (EMR) or trainable mentally retarded (TMR). The division for the two was based on IQ level, with the EMR group having an IQ of 50 or more. That classification determined where you went to school. The EMR students had a chance of being in a segregated classroom in a regular school in the district. The TMR students were sent outside the district to "special" schools where they could supposedly get the intensive services they needed. These schools were segregated and very often not the best of environments.

Sharon told me all this, so I knew the repercussions of a report from a psychologist saying Cindy would never have an IQ of more than 50. I was determined to keep her out of those segregated schools. However, despite all our efforts, Cindy ended up being placed in a segregated school run by the BOCES (Board of Cooperative Educational Services), a consortium of school districts. DeVillo Sloan was one of those segregated schools where most of the students were classified in the "trainable" category. Many students had severe cognitive and severe physical disabilities. After some investigation, I found out that the plan was to place my six-year-old daughter in a class of older, mostly male teenagers.

This began my education in the legal rights of students in the educational system. What I found out is that because she was classified as multiply handicapped, there was no age limit to the class groupings. They legally could do that. I was told they were trying to get more students so they could start a younger class, but if they were not successful, then she would be put in the older class. Everyone agreed this was not appropriate, but there was nothing I could do about it. I even contacted the New York State Department of Education's Regional Associate, and he told me they were within their rights. Had she been classified as only mentally retarded or physically disabled, there were age-range limitations to the class groupings. Once again, a single label attached to Cindy was impacting the direction of her life.

OFF TO A ROUGH START

Fortunately, two other younger students were enrolled, so the three students including Cindy were put into a separate class, and a teacher for the deaf was hired. I was so nervous and uncomfortable about the placement that I put Cindy on the bus the first day and then followed it to the school. I hid behind a bush so I could watch her get off the bus and go in. I had done the same thing her first day at the CP Center. I did it partly because I was nervous and protective and partly because I wanted to experience the thrill of a new milestone.

Her bus sat for a while, and finally the door opened and the students got out. The school was not officially open yet, so the students just lingered outside and the bus left. I stood there and observed my six-year-old deaf daughter standing pretty much alone on the sidewalk of this strange school not having any idea of where to go or what to do. She did not know anyone, no one knew her, and she looked confused and lost. There were no adults in sight. I was livid and immediately went to her and grabbed her hand. We went to the door and were told the students could not come in for another few minutes. I demanded to be let in and see the principal immediately. I was told he was not there as it was a religious holiday for him. I told the staff it was inappropriate to allow these students to wait outside unsupervised and I would deliver her myself to her class and speak to the principal the next day when he returned. I did just that, as well as contacted my district's transportation department to inform them of what happened. After a not-so-pleasant conversation with the principal, he agreed they would coordinate the buses better. I definitely was off to a rocky start at this school and had begun to establish my reputation as a troublemaker. So much for the thrill of the new milestone.

The school left a great deal to be desired, and the principal had, in my opinion, some very strange ideas. He was very keen on somewhat offbeat methods of therapy, including "swing therapy" where the students were put on large, flat swings for very long periods of time, sometimes hours. We did not see eye to eye on many issues and always seemed to be at odds with each other. I did not feel Cindy belonged at this school. I felt she was much smarter than most of the students and would not get enough stimulation. It was a depressing place, and I hated going there. I don't think Cindy liked it any better than I did. And Cindy always seemed happier and did better when she was around other children who did not have disabilities.

Despite the difficulties, the first year she was there, she had a wonderful teacher with a dual certification in special education and deaf education. During that first year with her, Cindy made wonderful progress, learning many new signs and developing this new method of communication. I was also taking sign language courses and learning how to communicate with her. Cindy seemed happy with her teacher and was progressing nicely. We had gone to the school district and requested that she be bussed after school to the day care center she had been attending. They were reluctant, and we had several meetings of what was then called the Committee on the Handicapped. I even got the NYS Department of Education's Regional Associate involved, and he attended an evening meeting of the committee, both very rare occurrences. After another battle over transportation, I got them to transport Cindy from school to the day care center. This allowed me to continue working full time.

At one time, part of that transportation was contracted to a private taxi company. I didn't think too much of this at the time but found out later that the driver was stopping at Burger King while Cindy was in the car. Besides this being what I thought was inappropriate, I felt it was also dangerous as he may have fed her something he should not have without knowing. Once again, I contacted the district's transportation department, and they called the taxi company and straightened it out. But the experience made me realize how vulnerable Cindy was and firmed my beliefs that secure safe transportation was essential.

I AM EXPECTING AGAIN

While Cindy was at the DeVillo Sloan school, I became pregnant again and was due in May 1979. Although we had been told that Cindy's problems were not genetic and there was no reason not to have more children, it took a long time for us to make that decision. We were afraid and tried to prepare ourselves for the worst. But in retrospect, I know we never truly believed it would happen again. Both Bob and I were happy and excited, as were our parents. We were looking forward to what every parent wants: a healthy child and all the hopes and dreams that go along with one. I had been working full time again for a few years, and Cindy was doing well with the teacher for the deaf.

Unfortunately, at about the five-month mark, I started having problems again. I was immediately put on total bed rest, and my employer put me on sick leave. This was very difficult for Bob as he not only had to take care of me but Cindy as well. He would get Cindy up and off to school in the morning, get me my breakfast, and make sure I had something for lunch, all before he went to work. He would pick up Cindy at daycare after work, bring her home, and make dinner for all of us. He had to do everything until I got the OK to get out of bed.

At about seven months, I was given more leeway if I did not overdo it. At about eight months, I began having contractions. The doctor started giving me shots and wanted Bob to continue them once a week at home so I wouldn't have to keep making the trip into the office. I wasn't sure Bob would do this as he would often come close to passing out when around needles, but the doctor assured me that he would be fine. Bob's mother commented to me that Bob would never be able to do that, but she was wrong too. He was quite good at it. Although he never hurt me, he constantly apologized in advance for doing so. The shots he gave me were easier than some I have had done by professionals. We both learned that we were much more capable than even we realized. Cindy had taught us that. She brought that out in us and showed us just how capable we really were.

It was during the latter part of my pregnancy that the teachers at Cindy's school embarked on an intensive toilet-training regime. Up until then nothing had been successful, and now with her newly acquired sign language and the use of a monitor attached to her leg, a strict regimen was started. I was now allowed out of bed and participated as much as physically possible. It was a lot for all of us to deal with at the time. However, Cindy responded extremely well and within a fairly short period of time she was successful. She was seven years old.

Deb was born on her due date using natural childbirth after an easy labor, and we thought we had a healthy child. All our dreams were coming true.

Cindy was thrilled to have a sister and smiled all the time at Deb. She loved to hold Deb and would often try to entertain her by offering her stuffed animals or other toys. Cindy would also watch me with Deb and offer help whenever she could.

CINDY HELPS DEB

Ironically, the knowledge that I had acquired from Cindy's experiences became my enemy. I knew much more about developmental milestones and normal development. I knew what should be happening and was watching closely. That knowledge quickly began to rob me of my hopes and dreams. They all crumbled ever so slowly and painfully.

Although Deb was a somewhat "colicky" baby due to issues with formula, the months after her birth were fairly typical. But because of my experiences with Cindy, I was now aware of developmental milestones. I began questioning her pediatricians at about five months. They felt we should keep a watchful eye for a few months. I felt in my gut that something was wrong, but few others seem to agree. I do not know if they didn't see any signs or just didn't want to see them. At eight months old, Deb was referred to the local Cerebral Palsy Center for evaluation. It was determined she had significant developmental delays but with no specific diagnosis. She was immediately enrolled in numerous therapies. Our lives instantly became more complicated. Once again, I found myself jockeying between therapies, doctor's appointments, and evaluations, in addition to seeking and evaluating appropriate programs for both girls. Working outside the home was no longer an option for me.

BUT SHE LOOKS SO NORMAL

Despite the many evaluations, it was still difficult for many to see Deb's problems. She was a beautiful baby, looked healthy with no obvious handicaps. Even Bob did not think we had anything to worry about.

One day a friend came to visit Bob and me in our home. He brought his granddaughter with him who was coincidentally about the same age as Deb. She was playing on the floor of our family room right alongside Deb as we all watched. As they played, I observed Bob looking back and forth between Deb and the other child. As he did, I could see the sudden realization of their differences expressed on his face. He now knew Deb had significant problems. His heart was breaking, and as I watched him, mine did too.

Although Deb did not have the physical abnormalities that Cindy did at birth, as it would turn out, her cognitive delays were more severe. But because of Cindy she got help early. I already knew how to navigate the system and where to go to get what she needed. If there was a silver lining to the dark cloud that was the discovery of her disabilities, it was Cindy. From medical issues to educational programs, Cindy helped Deb in so many ways without ever knowing it.

BEING CAREFUL ABOUT DEB'S LABELS

Because of my experiences with Cindy and labels, I was very cautious with Deb. I made sure any label would only help her and not pose an unwanted restriction. When Deb was approaching school age, the Committee on the Handicapped (COH) met to discuss placement. Deb was given the label of mentally retarded. They no longer broke it down like they did with Cindy. When the COH discussed placement and suggested DeVillo Sloan, my response was a loud and firm "over my dead body." It took some advocacy, but I kept her out of that segregated program. Although she was in a self-contained special education classroom, it was in a typical elementary school.

When Deb was seven years old, she was diagnosed with a seizure disorder. The neurologist that saw her on a regular basis asked if we had undergone genetic counseling. Although Deb's and Cindy's disabilities were different, the doctor was looking for a common thread. She suggested that we travel to a doctor in another state who may be able to determine whether they both fell into a common syndrome. I told her the story of our experience with the geneticist and asked what seeing another would buy us. Deb was getting everything she needed. I did not care about her having a label or putting a name on her problems. They could call it anything they wanted; it did not change anything. We would continue to make sure she got everything she needed. And I did not want to run the risk of a label hurting her like it did Cindy. We chose not to pursue it and the doctor did not push it. To this day we do not have a specific diagnosis. We have no specific cause or reason and therefore there is no blame. Deb is Deb and we see that she gets whatever she needs. We love her unconditionally. She is smart and a delight to be around.

ONCE AGAIN THERE WAS A MISTAKE

Cindy did so well the first year in the BOCES school that we decided to return to the psychologist specializing in the deaf for a follow-up. Cindy had had the benefit of the teacher for the deaf for a year and that made a big difference. Cindy was very cooperative and happy during the testing, which surprised the doctor. This time she was able to get some concrete results. She told us she was amazed at the difference in Cindy and told us she had made a mistake in her previous opinion. Her opinion now was that Cindy was functioning much higher than she previously had thought and was probably of borderline to low average intelligence. There were those words again, "I've made a terrible mistake." They were becoming all too familiar. But once again Cindy proved herself. And it had become my job to make sure she had the opportunity to do so. I was spending a great deal of time and effort making sure she had all the opportunities available. I knew Cindy was capable of more than people were saying and I was going to make sure she had the chance to show it. The professionals didn't listen to me, but they had to listen to Cindy.

The psychologist attributed Cindy's progress to the total communication approach and encouraged us to build on that and praised her teacher who was with us during the testing. Once again, Cindy had been misjudged and misdiagnosed but fortunately this time it did not impact her life as before. But Cindy, once again, taught the professional an important lesson.

A STEP BACKWARD

Unfortunately, Cindy's teacher had some serious issues with the school and the principal and because of them was leaving her position. When she did, there was no replacement, and I hounded not only the principal but also my school district and the state education department to do something about it. Somewhere I had lost that fear of speaking up and had become downright assertive. The old Cheryl did not exist anymore, and I could be as vocal as necessary. Cindy needed something and I was going to get it for her. Despite my efforts, I was not successful. The school was not able to find another teacher for the deaf, and Cindy was suffering because of it. She was put into a classroom of students who had very severe disabilities but were not deaf. Many had medical issues and needed a great deal of one-on-one for feeding and other daily living skills. Cindy functioned at a much higher level and really did not belong at the school at all. The recent evaluation from the psychologist supported our belief. Cindy wandered whenever she could to different classrooms, looking for other students to interact with. It became quite clear this was not an appropriate placement for her. So with the help of Sharon, the educational consultant, we set out to find a better one.

LOOKING FOR A BETTER PROGRAM

Our local school district had no program for students who were deaf but instead sent them to a BOCES program in another district or to a state-operated school. Sharon and I together looked at the local BOCES program for the deaf. It was housed in a typical elementary school, it had an excellent reputation, and we thought it would have been great for Cindy. However, they refused to accept Cindy because she had multiple disabilities, she was way behind academically, and they felt she would not fit well into their program. In addition, Cindy was receiving both physical therapy and occupational therapy, and neither was available in the school. We also looked at other local programs, some considerably smaller and some out of the county, but none would accept her. We could not find anything else locally that would provide her with what she needed — a total communication approach with a teacher for the deaf.

We investigated the New York State School for the Deaf in Rome, New York. They had a program for students with multiple handicaps, but it consisted of older students. They did, however, tell us they wanted to start another class of younger students but did not have enough students to support hiring a teacher. Cindy coming to their school would certainly help that. The school was very nice, and the staff we met seemed very good. Cindy could possibly be a day student, which would mean a long time on the bus every day, or she could be a residential student. They preferred that she spend at least one or two nights there for the socialization aspects. Although the school could provide what she needed academically, it was still a segregated school, and we were hesitant about that. We knew, however, that we had little choice, as the only local option was to continue in her current program, which was wrong for her. We began more and more to think about a school for the deaf, and I once again called on the school board parent. He encouraged me to investigate all the state schools and that is what I did.

The school in Rochester did not have any program for students with multiple disabilities, but the one in Buffalo did. We decided to visit and found that they had many years of experience with a multiple-handicapped program, and we liked what we saw. Everyone at the school was fluent in sign language, and she would have socialization with other deaf students. Cindy would of course have to be a residential student but would return home every weekend and all holidays, vacations, and all summer. It was a very difficult decision, but we felt we had no choice and we really didn't. At that time, inclusion or "mainstreaming," as it was referred to then, was just not being done to any great extent. Our choice was either DeVillo Sloan or a school for the deaf.

A formal application needed to be completed by us requesting placement, and typically the school closest to the student's home was the one the state approved. But we were leery of putting her in a program that wasn't sure they had enough students for a classroom and had no teacher we could meet or talk with beforehand. So when we applied to the state, we specifically requested St. Mary's in Buffalo and stated our reasons why. When the folks at the Rome school found out about it, they tried to block it and get the state to assign Cindy to them. I spoke with the people in Albany directly, explaining my reasons for requesting Buffalo. Cindy was going to have to be a residential student at either school, and I argued that I wanted the school I felt was the best match for her, one with a program already in existence with a record of accomplishment. Fortunately, the state agreed, and despite the arguments from the Rome school, Cindy's placement at St. Mary's School for the Deaf in Buffalo was approved.

At eight years old, Cindy would turn out to be St. Mary's youngest resident. We returned to Buffalo for the intake process, which included audiological testing, psychological testing, and the usual social history. We were also offered an opportunity to participate in what they called Family Learning Vacation. For a week in the summer, families stayed at the school with their child and participated in classes and activities.

Bob was unable to go for an entire week because of work, as well as the lack of someone to care for Deb that long. But Cindy and I went for the whole week, and Bob joined us on Friday night until Sunday while my parents took care of Deb. It was the most incredible week, and at the end of it, I knew for certain we had made the right decision. During the week there were many classes, and the entire time we were immersed in sign language. My skills improved dramatically. I learned so much about the deaf and developed wonderful relationships with some of the staff at the school. The group went on several outings and out for dinner. It was a wonderful week, and Cindy and I and Bob had a great time as well as learned a lot. It really made the separation that was looming somewhat easier.

Chapter 5
THE SCHOOL FOR THE DEAF

As September approached, Bob and I dreaded more and more the thought of Cindy living so far from home. We did not even know if we would be able to stand it but knew we had no choice. When the time came, we were nervous, and I didn't know how Cindy would react, although she seemed excited about going there. We decided that I would drive her up, spend some time talking with the residential staff, and put her to bed the first night. I wanted to be sure they knew how to care for her artificial leg, among other things. I was so concerned because there were so many things I wanted them to know; I sent a notebook that I had prepared with all the information in it. After all, Cindy could not communicate these things to them, so I had to do it for her. I remember the residential director telling me that usually she just got new students without parents. Sometimes new students would come in with their parents, but this was the first time a new student ever came with a book about them and she loved it. It contained some medical history, educational history, personal care instructions, a list of signs Cindy knew, and even foods she liked and didn't like. The residential department for the youngest students was very homey, with its own kitchen and sleeping and eating areas. The woman who supervised it was a lovely person who gave it a very family-like touch. There were only a few students, so Cindy received lots of attention. She even managed to conquer the training of her bowel movements. At eight years old, Cindy was finally completely toilet trained.

I spent that first afternoon and evening with Cindy at the school and put her to bed that night. I stayed in a motel and returned to get her up in the morning. I stuck around the following day and met most of the people who would be working with her during the day. I left that afternoon and returned home alone. The ride back seemed so strange and lonely, but because it was a short week, Cindy would be returning home the next day.

Even though the placement was approved by the state, it was also necessary for the school district to have a formal meeting of the Committee on the Handicapped (COH) and complete the recommendation. This committee is required to complete an individualized education plan (IEP), which formally designates her program and services. Once approved, the district is bound to those services until they are formally changed. The district was mandated to provide transportation to and from the school, a three-hour ride that they contracted out to a private company. I had asked if Cindy could go on Monday morning but was told by the school that they felt she would lose too much and recommended she come on Sunday. I convinced the school district to arrange her transportation so she could spend as much time as possible at home. I was told that the transportation company wanted to pick Cindy up at 1:00 in the afternoon and I felt that was too early. We managed to get it changed so she wouldn't leave until 5:00 p.m. At least that way we could have an early dinner with her, and she wouldn't get to Buffalo terribly late.

Cindy seemed very happy about her new school and had done well those first few days. A communication book came home as it would every week so that we could write back and forth with both the teacher and the residential staff. I still have all those books, and many years after she first went to the school, the original notebook I sent was returned to me as well.

IT WAS SO HARD FOR US

When it came time to send Cindy back that first weekend, it was much harder than we expected. Even though Cindy was happy and left without any problems, Bob and I were devastated. When she was picked up, we waved goodbye, told her we loved her, then we both came back inside put our arms around each other and cried. She was only eight years old and to us still a baby. We could not believe we were sending her away. It was so very difficult and would remain so for a very long time. It was many weeks before we could send her off without crying after she left.

The academic part of the program was very good, and she had a terrific teacher. The class was composed of only five or six students who floated in and out for other activities or therapies. The students got a good deal of individual attention. Cindy and the others wore a Phonic Ear hearing aid system that worked with the teacher's unit, which she controlled to allow sound from her alone or to include background. The only problem I had with the class was that it was located in the basement and was the only classroom down there. I was told it was that way because the students were easily distracted and the atmosphere was quieter. While I understood that and appreciated it, I pointed out to both the teacher and the administration that I thought that separating them from the rest of the students was detrimental and sent a negative message. I don't know if my comments had any influence or not, but the class was moved upstairs the next year.

I visited school as often as I could and would sometimes stay overnight to take Cindy out to dinner or attend some school function. Bob and I both went up to watch their annual gym show that first year. Cindy wore white leotards with red tights and looked adorable. The gym was filled with the usual mats, swings, and bars, and we wondered what equipment she would be able to use with her artificial leg. We watched her as she bounced with a teacher on the trampoline and were amazed when she did a routine on the uneven parallel bars. She was happy and beaming from ear to ear. Bob and I were so proud of her.

FINDING A SUMMER PROGRAM

Because there was no program in the summer, we wanted to find something for Cindy to do to keep her busy. We also did not want her to lose the progress she had made during the school year. There was a program run by the association for the deaf that was housed at a typical day camp. It would provide the necessary educational components as well as speech therapy and was approved by the state as a summer program. It would be great for Cindy and would be fun too. But first I had to get them to accept her, and they were reluctant to do so. The area where the program was located was very hilly and would involve a good deal of walking. They didn't feel Cindy could handle the terrain with her artificial leg. I really think they just plain didn't want her in the program, but the only reason they gave me was mobility. After much persistence, I finally convinced them to consider her. They agreed provided they could do a test. The director of the program wanted Cindy to visit the site and walk around with her. I think she was convinced Cindy would not be able to handle it. Cindy and I met her there, and she walked the both of us all over the site, including hills and trails. I was exhausted but Cindy did just fine, much to the director's surprise. Because the mobility issue was the only reason given for not accepting her, when Cindy did so well, the program had to agree to take her. Cindy attended that camp for many summers and enjoyed it immensely.

MOVING UP

The second year at St. Mary's, Cindy transferred to the Junior Girls residential department. The director of this department was a nun. Despite the name of the school and the presence of nuns, the school is not religion-based and cannot be because it is funded with public money. Nevertheless, the influence was there. Sister ran her department with a very tight grip. The room where the girls slept was dormitory style, and every bed looked exactly the same. Each bed had identical bedspreads with a stuffed animal on it and identical chairs sitting to the right of each bed. It was all very uniform. I hated that part of the school, and over time, it would prove to be detrimental to Cindy as well.

Although Cindy was eager to go back to school in the fall, shortly after, she started protesting when it was time to go. We were not sure what was going on so once again, I turned to the parent whose daughter went to St. Mary's. He spoke with his daughter, and she told him it was not unusual when the girls first came to this department to have some difficulty adjusting. This was a much larger group, girls only, and was much more regimented. Schedules and routines were strictly adhered to. There were twenty or so girls in the residential department, so they didn't get the individual attention from the staff but they did have each other. We gave it a bit of time and after a while Cindy calmed down. But for quite a while, she cried when it was time to return to school. That made sending her back so very difficult for Bob and me. We did whatever we could to make things better for her, and when she was home, we did special things just with her. We always felt guilty that she was gone during the week. Deb had us all to herself then, and we spent a great deal of time with her and therapies and programs. So we made a point of doing things with just Cindy on weekends and vacations that did not include Deb. We called it her "special time" and even took her on "special vacations." Of course, we had family time also.

One "special vacation" we took just before Cindy was to return to school at the end of a summer. While we were away, we stopped at a shoe store and bought her a new pair of shoes for school. A couple of years later, again at the end of summer, we were on a similar trip although not in the same place. We spent a few days in Lake George, New York, and had a wonderful time together. We took a boat ride on the lake and a carriage ride around the town and saw all the local tourist spots. Cindy had fun swimming in the motel's pool and really enjoyed eating out. It was a terrific vacation.

Before heading home, we stopped at a shopping center to look for new shoes for Cindy. We were not able to find anything and started to leave. Cindy started acting out, grabbing shoes, and throwing them, grabbing at us, and trying to pull down displays. It was awful, and we struggled to get her out of the store. We could not understand what was wrong with her. We started to drive home, and Cindy was sitting in the back seat as she always did. Cindy was clearly still upset although calmer than before. We had done all we thought we could when Cindy suddenly opened the car door while Bob was driving on the highway at 60 mph. Despite our efforts to get her to stop, she continued to do it. Unfortunately, our car did not have child safety locks or power locks. So I rode the entire way home sitting next to her in the backseat, ready to stop her from opening the door again. It was a long and uncomfortable three-hour ride back. During that time, we remembered that twice before when on a vacation we had bought a pair of shoes for her.

It was now so evident how much of an influence her routines had on her. If she did something more than once, she thought that was the way it always should be. It was our first inclination of the effect of the strict regimen at St. Mary's. This proved to be very problematic and posed tremendous problems for us for many years. She was also showing us that she was smart enough to know how to get our attention. When she did not get what she wanted by the temper tantrum in the store, she upped the ante. We will never know if she got angry because she didn't get shoes or because she knew she would be returning to school or something entirely different. To this day, we need to be careful about routines. Cindy still can have difficulty accepting change, although she is definitely more flexible than she was during her time at St. Mary's.

We did not always know what would upset Cindy or when it would happen and still don't. Once while she was home from school for the weekend, we took her to a Syracuse University vs. Notre Dame basketball game. Bob and I had season tickets, and we felt guilty going out on her night at home. She had gone to games with us before and enjoyed it. We bought an extra ticket and used the special transportation provided by the university. They had a handicapped parking lot with a bus that dropped you off at the door of the Dome so there was very little walking. Cindy was very excited and seemed to be enjoying herself. During the halftime of what was a terrific game, she kept looking behind us. Our seats were in the last row of the second deck with the hallway right behind us, and it was filled with people getting refreshments. Cindy continued to look back and became increasingly more upset. Despite our efforts to redirect her and calm her down, she became increasingly agitated until she started to grab at the people sitting in front of us. We were unable to determine the cause of her upset and unable to stop her from grabbing so we finally had to get her out of the seats. We couldn't get a bus back to our car yet as it was only the beginning of the second half. So the three of us stood in the basement hallway watching one of the most exciting games in Syracuse history on the TV monitor. Cindy was fine after she left the seats, and we never knew what it was that upset her so much.

These kinds of problems did not deter us from doing things with Cindy. We took her on many outings and vacations both alone and with Deb and we had many wonderful times. Despite everything she had been through, Cindy was still a happy child who smiled almost all the time.

Cheryl Kantak

CINDY IS TRYING TO TELL US SOMETHING

During her second year in the Junior Girls Department, I noticed that when Cindy came home on the weekends, she was having very large and hard bowel movements. I asked Sister if this was a problem at school, and she told me she was concerned because Cindy was not having any bowel movements so she had asked for the physician to see her. They sent her to a local neurologist, and he in turn sent her for an EEG. I never understood why an EEG was ordered for constipation, but the report came back indicating no evidence of epileptic activity and no further recommendations.

Cindy started on a regimen of receiving a suppository from the nurse on a regular basis while she was at school. Although this solved the problem temporarily, it still did not determine the cause so I made a visit. I spoke with a lot of people and determined that Cindy seemed to be doing well in class so that wasn't an issue. After speaking with Sister in the residential department, I found out that Cindy was no longer going to the local college to swim once a week with the other girls as she had been. I knew this was something Cindy loved so I asked why. I was told she had an accident in the pool and had to be taken out immediately. I asked if Cindy was punished for the accident in some way, and Sister told me no. However, Cindy was not allowed to swim again. Sister told me she couldn't jeopardize the other girls losing access to the pool. Sister assured me a big deal was not made of the accident, but I think differently. In my opinion, the experience must have traumatized Cindy because it was right after it happened that she started withholding her bowel movements. I tried to make Sister understand that Cindy was being punished, but she didn't see it that way.

When Cindy returned home for the summer, everything would return to normal, but when she went back to school, it would start all over again and she would once again need suppositories. I made many trips to school to try to work out some of these issues with

Sister. At one time I suggested that perhaps Cindy could have a commode beside her bed in case she needed to go to the bathroom during the night. Sister refused as she felt it would not be fair to the other girls if one girl had something they didn't. I could not make her understand even when I reminded her that Cindy did not wear her artificial leg in bed and could not walk to the bathroom like everyone else. Sister was older and very set in her ways and would not budge. Everything had to be uniform no matter what the circumstances.

We hated the residential part of the school. I frequently went to meetings and conferences there and voiced my concerns. It wasn't an awful place but, in my view, it was very institutional and had the effects of an institution. Cindy was told when to go to the bathroom. Showers or routines were done at the time it fit into Sister's schedule. Someone even followed Cindy into the bathroom and stood by the opened stall door to make sure she went. It was so regimented that it robbed Cindy of her individuality, and she waited to be told or given permission to do everything; that influence haunts her to this day. We constantly struggled with this negative part of the school, weighing it against the academic part that was so good for Cindy. The good side to the residential department was that Cindy had other deaf girls to socialize with. She even joined the Girl Scouts and went on occasional outings with them.

RELIABLE TRANSPORTATION IS A MUST

Transportation continued to be an issue. Our school district contracted that out to a private company. The man who ran it would pick Cindy up and drop her off in a Suburban van. He started down around the Utica area and had several students, including some who were both deaf and blind. Bob and I became concerned because he was the only adult in the vehicle with seven or eight students and Cindy was the only female. We worried about the possibility of something happening and also wondered what he would do if Cindy had to use the restroom. We certainly didn't want her wandering in a Thruway stop by herself. I asked if he could get someone else to go with him. He did so on occasion but not often. So I went again to the school district and requested that her transportation include a female aide on the bus. They agreed and for a while there was a female on the van. However, it happened more and more that she would not be there. When I inquired, I was told he had no substitute. He jokingly asked if I wanted to do it and I said I would. So, when he came with no aide, I would ride up to the school with him and he would drop me off on his way back home. Of course, I was not paid for my time but it was a real learning experience. I was able to casually get information I never had before.

One time he stopped at a rest area, pulled up in front of the door, and got out to get a cup of coffee and probably go to the men's room. I sat in the car with the students. When he returned, I asked what he did when he didn't have an aide and he told me he just locked the doors. After that, I made sure he always had an aide in the car or I went with him. The van was full of students who were deaf, blind, or both, and all had very little or no communication skills. Cindy was so vulnerable and so many things could happen.

ONE SCARY NIGHT

This was never more evident than one snowy Sunday night. We had made a habit of checking the Thruway weather reports, and this night, although it was snowy, everything was open. About an hour after Cindy was picked up, we received a call from Sister at the school telling us it was snowing very hard and perhaps Cindy shouldn't come. I explained she had already left, and we agreed to contact one another if we heard anything. It normally took them about three-and-a-half hours to get to the school as they stopped at the Batavia School for the Blind to drop students off there. Normally they should have been in Buffalo between 8:00 and 9:00 p.m. After we got that call from school, we continued to check the Thruway reports and found out later they had shut down the western part of it. We checked in with school a couple of times, and at 10:00 p.m., there was still no word. The Batavia school had not heard from them either. We were frantic and did not know what to do. Bob and I were both pacing the floor, sick with worry. We were considering calling the State Police to see if they could help us when close to 11:00 p.m. we got a call that they were at the school for the blind in Batavia. They had to leave the Thruway when it closed and were forced to take the back roads. One of the staff got on the phone and told me that Cindy was fine, and they would be staying there until the storm was over. I was assured she was going to be well cared for and would be given everything she needed. Boy were we relieved and grateful they had made it that far and weren't on the side of the road someplace or worse. The experience cemented in my mind the importance of safe and reliable transportation.

WE CANNOT LET THIS GO ON

Over time, the safety issue became more of a concern for us as we noticed the vehicle being used was deteriorating. I had established a good relationship with the driver/owner of the company. When I casually mentioned I was surprised the vehicle passed inspection, he smiled and said he had a friend who took care of it. Bob and I became concerned when we would see things like broken taillights week after week, heavily worn tires, and holes due to excessive rusting.

We also started to get the feeling that something else was going on. After several years of the same transportation, we were used to seeing the same kids, and I paid close attention to who was in the vehicle when she was picked up and dropped off. I am not exactly sure why or how I thought something was fishy but I knew something was not right. When I asked questions of the driver, he seemed reluctant to give answers. I was seeing different students at times and sometimes more students than usual. I contacted my school district transportation department and told them my concerns, both about the number of students in the van and the condition of it. They said they would do some checking and indeed found out they were making another stop after us and picking up more students from a different area.

The school district contacted the NYS Department of Transportation (DOT) and a representative called me. I explained my concerns, and he asked what time Cindy was picked up. He stopped by our house on a Sunday afternoon and asked what route the van usually took when it left our house. We gave all the information he requested, then he thanked us and left. Of course, we never said anything to the driver but suspected the DOT was going to check up on him.

We found out later that week that the DOT representative was waiting when they got on the Thruway. They pulled him over and cited him for numerous safety violations. That prompted a further investigation that uncovered he was overloading the vehicle with students, which prompted more citations. When Cindy came back that Friday, the driver/owner was in a lousy mood and told us what had happened. He said he was sure someone blew him in and it was not random. Of course, we did not want his anger to be taken out on Cindy so we played dumb. It was all very cloak and dagger, and I worried what would happen if he found out it was us. I didn't have to worry about it very long because the school district terminated his contract and hired someone else.

ANOTHER AMPUTATION

When Cindy was 12 years old, she had grown tall enough that her artificial leg became a problem. All the painful surgery and aftermath of it turned out to be for nothing. The efforts to save the lower part of her leg did not work; Cindy had a prosthesis that did not bend. Although she had no problem walking with it that way, when she would sit down, her leg had to be straight out. The taller she got, the more cumbersome that became, and even riding in the car became difficult. She could only ride in the front seat where we could put the seat back and there was more leg room or she had to sit sideways in the back. If she went to the movies, she had to sit in the end seat with her leg in the aisle. It would be the same as if someone had a full-length cast on their leg.

We knew we would have to do something about this and that it would necessitate further surgery. We were so reluctant to do that because we had just gotten Cindy to the point where we could take her places easily and we did not want to traumatize her again with another hospitalization.

She had a different orthopedic doctor by now, and when we spoke to him about it, he advised us to have more surgery. However, he also told us that he wanted to try a different procedure on her that he thought would help. When I inquired as to what he wanted to do, he became defensive and told me to leave the medical issues to him. This had an all-too-familiar ring, and I quite frankly did not like his attitude so I asked our pediatrician to refer us to someone else. This time I wanted to go somewhere that was well-known and had a good deal of experience with this type of thing. Someone had mentioned to me the Ontario Crippled Children's Hospital in Toronto, so I wrote them about Cindy and her situation. They said they would be glad to see her but that I needed a referral from her doctor as well as her records. After some work with our local doctors, we got an appointment and were offered a place to stay overnight. They had a small motel on the premises that they used for patients and families. We gratefully accepted and made the arrangements.

Cheryl Kantak

A SECOND OPINION

When we crossed the border into Canada, we were, of course, asked where we were going and the purpose of our visit. Being honest, we told them exactly why we were there, after which we were instructed to pull over to the building. Bob had to go in and answer more questions. There really was no problem, but they were being cautious as apparently many people had entered the country on the same premise and then attempted to stay beyond that. They were very nice and told us we were going to one of the finest places we could possibly have chosen. They were right on target.

Our appointment was the next day, so we checked into the motel for the night. Cindy became extremely upset and cried and fussed and acted out the entire night. We had a terrible time calming her down, and none of us got much sleep. We worried she would be so uncooperative that the trip would be for nothing. I do not know what upset her, but the next day when we went to the center, she could not have been better.

The doctors and staff there were incredibly nice and were gentle and compassionate while they did their exams and took their information. This was a place where many people came for appointments or therapies, and they asked if we would like to meet some of the patients. We agreed and were introduced to a lovely young woman in her teens. She had the exact same defect in her leg that Cindy had, only she had it in both legs. Both her legs were amputated above the knee, and she had two full leg prostheses. When we first met her, she was wearing both legs but later she took them off. Cindy's eyes nearly bulged out of her head when she realized this girl was like her. The other girl was so warm and kind and understanding, and they bonded instantly. We thanked her profusely and spoke again with the doctors. Their advice was to revise Cindy's amputation to an above-the-knee one and not to do any more experimental surgery. I think we had already made up our minds to take that route, but hearing their recommendation certainly solidified our decision. We asked if they could recommend a doctor in our area and they gave us a name.

WHAT A DIFFERENCE A DOCTOR CAN MAKE

Bob and I both took Cindy to see the orthopedic doctor who was at the same teaching hospital as her first one, so we were very leery. But after meeting him, we were confident he was the right one. He absolutely agreed there should be no further experimentation. He assured us he would do everything he could to reduce the trauma to Cindy. We talked about several things we could do, including making a pre-visit to the hospital and specific floor to meet the nurses and explain everything to Cindy beforehand. He helped us arrange all that, and Cindy responded well to it.

Previously, we had made a visit to the place that made her prosthesis, where she was shown what a new leg with a bendable knee would look like. She was very excited about the prospect of a new leg that would bend, and we explained that first she would need to go into the hospital. Jean, Cindy's teacher from St. Mary's, also worked with us and made Cindy's upcoming surgery a discussion in class as something that was exciting and would help her. We did not lie to Cindy and told her there would be "hurt" and therapy, and she would be out of school for a couple of months. Because of that we arranged through the school district to have homebound teaching during that time. Jean came to visit her and met with the homebound teacher and brought school work. We spent a great deal of time preparing Cindy and just hoped for the best.

The surgery went well and the doctor was wonderful. Cindy had a difficult time post-op and was doing a lot of vomiting and grabbing at people. Even though some discomfort was expected, I felt there was something else wrong again but I couldn't quite put my finger on it. I thought the pain medication might be the cause of her distress and suggested it be stopped. One of the nurses yelled at me and told me Cindy could not possibly tolerate the pain. I told her Cindy had a high pain tolerance, she was clearly not comfortable now, and I wanted to give it a try. The nurse looked at me like I was the worst mother on the face of the earth. I felt a little like the wicked witch of the North. I spoke with the doctor and told him I had a hunch the pain medication was making her sick and I wanted to stop it. Fortunately, he agreed with me and we stopped the pain medicine. The vomiting stopped, Cindy's mood improved dramatically, and although I am sure she was uncomfortable, she looked and acted considerably better.

Bob and I took turns staying with her overnight, and the next day when the doctor came to see her, he suggested we would probably be better off at home. He gave me specific things to do and look for, as well as his home phone number if I had any problems. He was truly a gem, and I believe partly because of him and his compassion and concern, Cindy came through the experience beautifully. Cindy once again showed the medical people they did not have all the answers.

After the initial healing period, Cindy was fitted with a new prosthesis with a bendable knee. She had physical therapy two to three times a week to help her learn how to walk with the new leg. Eventually, she learned how to walk bending the knee but often reverted to the stiff leg. We tried to encourage her to walk normally but she was off balance and obviously felt insecure. Over time, she continued not to use the prosthesis as it was intended and only bent the knee when she sat down. I spoke with her doctor about it, and he advised us not to force her. He felt that she had learned to walk with a stiff leg and had used it that way for so long that she probably felt too unsteady walking with it bent. She had the capability to bend the leg when necessary, and he assured me it would not be harmful in any way for her to keep it straight when she walked.

Cindy was showing us once again that she had a mind of her own and she was very capable of making her own decision about this. While I think she was grateful she had the ability to bend the knee when she sat, she definitely wanted it stiff when she walked. All our preparation paid off because Cindy not only came through the whole thing without reverting to her previous insecurity but also seemed to enjoy all the attention. In fact, after that, she loved going to the doctor and rarely acted up during appointments. Even now she is great going to the doctor as long as they aren't doing something new to her.

A STRONG MESSAGE FROM CINDY

When Cindy was fourteen years old, she moved up to the Senior Girls' residential department at St. Mary's. This department was also supervised by a nun, but she was much different than the previous one. The routine in this residential department was much less structured and allowed for much more individuality. It took Cindy a while to acclimate herself to this different setting but eventually she really liked it. She had to get used to being able to do things without waiting to be told and eventually she did just that. However, to this day, she easily falls back to waiting for a prompt to do something.

After moving to this residential department, she also no longer needed the suppository. That was a strong statement to us that she had clearly been unhappy in the other department, and the withholding of her bowel movements was a sign of distress and a form of communication. It was a lesson we never forgot and one that would be repeated years later.

WHAT ABOUT THE FUTURE?

While the newer residential setting was better, it still left a great deal to be desired. As Cindy became older, I began to think more and more about the future. I thought about what would happen when she was no longer in school. What would she do and where would she live?

I had become knowledgeable in the special education field by attending workshops and conferences and by being the parent member of my district's Committee on the Handicapped (COH). I had taken a part-time job with a Parent Training Project, a federally funded program. As part of that job, I did a great deal of advocacy work with other parents, helping them to get special education services for their children. I also conducted numerous workshops all around New York State on the educational rights of students with disabilities as well as communication and advocacy skills. Thanks to Cindy, presenting in front of a group was no longer a problem for me. The project also helped parents with the transition from school to adult services. Through my work, I was able to attend other conferences in the field and tap many resources. The result was I became knowledgeable in the field. So I started to ask a lot of questions at school.

"Do the older students have a job outside of school?" At that time, they did not.

"Do they date?" I asked.

"No, they are not allowed to date. They are not equipped to deal with rejection, but we do have supervised dances and parties."

"I do not take rejection well either. I am sure when they leave school, they do not suddenly become equipped," I replied.

I became more and more aware of how sheltered the school was and worried about what would happen when Cindy "graduated." She would have to live and function in a hearing world and keeping her from that now was not going to help. Academically, it had become obvious she would not graduate with a regular diploma and would have serious academic deficiencies. She still could not read or write. So now our focus needed to be on preparing her for the real world; St. Mary's was not the real world. This was a place where the boys and girls still used separate stairways and walked single file through the halls, even in high school. I always thought she was protected there but that wasn't preparing her for the years that followed. They had no vocational component to their high school program for students labeled "multiply handicapped," and Cindy needed the vocational training. So I began to work on bringing her back home.

I knew the director of special education in our district well and saw her frequently when the committee I was on would meet. I had also worked closely with her when Deb reached school age. I made sure that Deb was in a district program. I did not want her to be segregated like Cindy was. I also got to know many of the other teachers, psychologists, and staff, from both my committee involvements and my job with the Parent Training Project. I began to talk with people in the district about bringing Cindy back to a local program. At her annual school district's review, they agreed to send a psychologist up to Buffalo to observe Cindy and assess her needs.

CINDY DOES NOT SEEM HAPPY AT SCHOOL

At about the same time, Cindy started to be less happy with St. Mary's. Although she was doing OK in the classroom, she was starting to act out at times in the residential department. A behavior consultant who periodically worked with the school was brought in and a plan devised. Martha was a wonderful woman and very talented. She consulted all over the country, specializing in behavior modification for students who were deaf. She worked with the school and us as well. One thing she liked to do each year, so she could, as she put it, "keep in touch," was to go to a family's home and spend some time with the children without the parents.

One year Martha offered to stay with both girls in our home while we went away for a few days. She did not charge to do this but considered it her training. As respite for us was nearly impossible to get, we jumped at the opportunity. We were so eager to get away that we went despite the fact I had a fractured knee and my leg was in a full-length hard cast. We left her with everything she would need and had a wonderful three days. This proved to be the start of a long-lasting friendship. She helped us enormously while Cindy was at St. Mary's and would prove later just what a good friend she was.

PREPARING FOR HER RETURN

We continued to talk with people in our local school district about the possibility of Cindy returning home and attending the local high school. She would of course need an interpreter and would be in a self-contained special education class. But the focus of her program would be to develop the life skills and training she would need after school.

Our high school's program was community-based; the students learned their skills outside of school and eventually were matched with a job. I spoke with the teacher whom I already knew. I also brought Cindy to her classroom and after a while left her there for a short time at the teacher's request. Cindy and I went to the school on another occasion to meet with the guidance counselor. The teacher also came to our home to observe Cindy and talk with us. I have always been open with teachers about Cindy and have never lied about her so I told her about her outbursts and how we handled them.

I asked the teacher if she would like to visit St. Mary's, and she said that was not necessary. I offered to bring the behavior specialist, Martha, to the school at my expense. She told me she was very familiar with behavior modification and that also was not necessary. I told her I would be glad to sign any necessary releases so that she could speak with Cindy's former teachers, but she declined that offer as well. She had many years of experience working with students with disabilities and felt quite capable of handling this. She agreed to take Cindy in her class; actually, this was not a requirement for placement, but we were trying to do this the right way by working cooperatively with everyone involved.

At the next annual meeting of the school district's committee, they formally approved Cindy's return to our high school. At that meeting, the psychologist who had visited St. Mary's mentioned there was a behavior plan in place there, and it was made a part of Cindy's IEP (individualized educational plan). It also specified she was to have a full-time interpreter for the deaf, as well as a consulting teacher for the deaf.

Although Cindy was very excited about the prospect of living at home again, the folks at St. Mary's had made it clear they thought we were making a terrible mistake. But despite their opposition, that June, eight years after she began, Cindy and I said our thank yous and goodbyes to all the people in Buffalo. It was a bittersweet time as we had so many wonderful friends and memories there. Change had always been scary for Cindy and for us, but this was a new beginning. We had just moved into a brand-new house we built with the girls' accessibility needs in mind, and Cindy was coming back home to live year-round. We were all very excited.

I have no doubt that Cindy has many fond memories of her time at St. Mary's. Whenever she is in the area, she always wants to visit the school.

Chapter 6
CINDY ATTENDS OUR LOCAL HIGH SCHOOL

Cindy was very excited to start school that fall. We had visited the school again during the summer and showed her around. I decided not to go to school the first couple of days because I felt it was a difficult time for teachers and students settling in, and they did not need a mom hanging around. I sent a notebook in with a note to both the teacher and the interpreter giving them some information and my offer of help if there was anything they needed.

PROBLEMS START

The first week went OK but shortly after that I received a call during the day to come and get Cindy. She had gotten angry and thrown a calculator across the room. When I arrived, she had been removed from the classroom and was sitting in an adjoining room with several adults. The teacher told me she would not tolerate that behavior and to take Cindy home and tell her she could not act like that again. I spoke with the interpreter and found out that she had not even assigned name signs to people. She had made little effort to learn about Cindy's needs and she was not a certified interpreter.

I repeated my offers of help from others, but they were flatly refused with a tone of being insulted by the offer.

The next day while on an outing to the shopping mall, Cindy acted out again when she was not allowed to purchase a poster. This was something she was used to doing, but the class had been told they were there only to look. Once again, she was sent home. Every time Cindy had any kind of outburst in the class, the teacher would call us to come get her. She also involved the school's principal and guidance counselor. Because we were still trying to work cooperatively with the school, we left a number whenever we went anywhere.

One time I was in a board meeting and could not be reached, so they called Bob's boss. Bob was working on a job about an hour away and was forced to drive back to get Cindy. When he arrived at the high school, Cindy was calmly sitting in a separate room with five adults. Cindy had acted out again by throwing something and grabbing a teacher. One of the administrative staff strongly stated that they did not have behavior problems in their school and they were not going to tolerate them now. Cindy was suspended from school for five days. Coincidentally, two days later, the school made the local newspaper's front-page headlines because of a massive fight that broke out between "typical" students on school property. It was major news in the papers and on the TV for several days. A few students were both arrested and expelled while others involved got away without even a one-day suspension. With all of this going on, Cindy throwing something or grabbing was considered to them to be unacceptable and grounds for removal. The irony did not escape us.

Bob and I and Sharon, our educational consultant, had numerous meetings with school personnel to try to rectify the situation. We did everything we could to help, as well as try to figure out what was causing the problem. During our meetings, it became obvious to us that the so-called interpreter was just a teaching assistant who had taken a couple of sign language courses. I observed her using incorrect signs and trying to change Cindy's signs. It is common for people who are deaf to have slightly different versions of a sign depending on where they were educated. She was unable to recognize some of Cindy's signs and was acting in roles other than an interpreter. And the consulting teacher for the deaf had not yet been contacted.

THEY REFUSE ALL HELP

We offered to bring in outside consultants to help. One such person, a PhD, was from a project associated with the School of Special Education at Syracuse University. She met with us and school personnel after the second incident. This project was designed to work with teachers and staff in classrooms where there were special education students with behavior difficulties. The assistance of these experts would have been provided free of charge to the district. The school refused their help. They were concerned the assistance was not enough and the results would take too long.

I also offered once again to bring the consultant from St. Mary's that had worked with Cindy to the school at my expense. That was also refused. It was clear very soon that the teacher did not want Cindy in that class and was not open to any suggestions. At one point she even said to the administration in front of us, "They created the problem; let them fix it."

Shortly after that meeting, while on a class field trip, Cindy acted out again. We learned later that the interpreter had been intentionally pulled away from Cindy by the teacher, supposedly to allow natural interaction. However, it also robbed her of her means of communicating as no one else knew sign language. When a problem developed with another student, once again, Cindy was sent home and suspended for two days.

The first day she was back, there was another incident while she was in gym class. Once again much later, the teacher involved testified she felt it was a communication problem. However, less than two months into the school year, Cindy was suspended from school, and a meeting was set up with the school superintendent. It was never clear if this meeting was a formal superintendent's hearing, but Sharon started consulting in the background with an advocate from our local legal services office. They advised we tape-record the meeting.

THE SUPERINTENDENT'S MEETING

Both Bob and I, with Sharon, attended the meeting, which was held in October, and we were only three against what seemed like the cast of *Ben Hur*. When the superintendent began the meeting, I asked if he had anyone taking notes. He replied it was not a formal hearing and therefore he didn't unless I wanted to make it a formal hearing. I explained that if no one had any objections I would like to tape-record the meeting so that I would have an accurate recollection. I stated it was easier for me than trying to take notes. I tried my best to say it in a way that was not threatening. I started the recorder and someone began speaking when the superintendent abruptly interrupted.

"Wait just a minute. I object to this. I have a reputation in this district for being a fair person and I find this very insulting. I want that turned off."

It was clear to me more than ever that it was needed, but keeping it on would do more harm than good. I apologized if I had insulted him as it was not my intent and removed the recorder from the table.

"I need a minute to compose myself," he said. With his elbows on the table and his head resting in his hands, he sat for well over a minute while everyone silently waited before he gave his permission to proceed. It was a performance worthy of an Oscar. The rest of the meeting was far less dramatic, not at all productive, and very tense. The outcome was that nothing was settled and no long-term solution was found. The Committee on the Handicapped was charged with finding a solution. We left the meeting knowing very little except that Cindy was not going to be back in the classroom until the situation could be reassessed.

There were several more meetings of the COH, and despite my requests to have Cindy back in school, they would not agree.

CINDY HAS NO PROGRAM

Cindy had no program for over a month until we pointed out they were in violation of law by not providing something. They finally recommended to give her homebound teaching in school six hours a week, her therapies and job training six hours a week, but no interaction with other students. We did not agree because we wanted a full-day program with other students. We also pointed out that the recommended program did not comply with NYS regulations. And it certainly was not the least restrictive environment.

Cindy had a difficult time with all of this and continued to ask to go to school. She would have tears in her eyes when she saw her sister, Deb, getting on and off the bus and clearly did not understand why she could not go too. She would cry and act out and all I could do was try to make her understand what was happening, but clearly, she did not. I told her over and over that Mom and Dad were doing everything we could to get her back in school.

Her homebound in-school was in a classroom with the homebound teacher, Veronica, the same teaching assistant or so-called interpreter, and Cindy. She had no contact with other students. It did not start until the end of October and was for only two hours a day, two days a week to start. I had to transport her back and forth. It just so happened that at the same time, the Parent Training Project I worked for part time had lost its funding, so I was out of a job. It was probably a good thing because there would have been no way I could have kept a job with what we were going through. After Cindy was placed in this very segregated environment, the school decided they would take the offer of help from the Syracuse University project. However, the terms of their grant would not allow them to work with students in such a segregated setting. They could only help if Cindy was in a classroom with other students. The timing of the school district's reconsideration was very interesting.

Cindy was happy to have something, but every time we went to school, we had to pass by her old classroom, and she would always stop and point to it indicating she wanted to go in. It broke my heart.

Veronica was hired specifically for this job and was a wonderful teacher. She had no experience with a student who was deaf but was enthusiastic and took all the help and advice she could get. Cindy liked her teaching assistant, and she was also cooperative. After a while, Cindy got some of her therapies as well, so I did a lot of transporting back and forth to school. At the end of November, she started in a job site for an hour a week, another service she was supposed to be receiving all along. Some services did not begin until the end of January and some not at all. Her schedule was so sporadic that I kept a calendar where I wrote down every service she got, never realizing at the time how important that would become later.

All this time we continued to work toward getting her back into the classroom, without success. Sharon and I both felt that the original teacher and the superintendent were working behind the scenes, putting pressure on people to keep that from happening. The director of special education whom I had worked with for so long, who knew me and helped me bring Cindy back, gave us the impression her hands were tied. At one meeting we made it clear that we were considering exercising our right of due process. After the meeting, while standing off to the side with Sharon, the director of special education came up to us and quietly said to us, "Go do what you have to do." It was clear to us she was on our side but was not being allowed to help at all.

TAKING THE LEGAL ROUTE

At this time, 1988, due process, or an impartial hearing as it was also called, was anything but impartial. A hearing could be formally requested by either the parent or the school district, but generally the family initiated it. After a formal request to the school board, a hearing officer was assigned from a list of approved people who mostly were other school district administrators. The school district gets to make the choice and pays their fee, hardly impartial, which is why for the most part parents do not prevail.

We were referred to our local Legal Services office, which also had a Protection and Advocacy program. Because of Cindy's disabilities, she qualified for their services, and they could represent her free of charge. They had a minimal number of attorneys so they only took a few select cases. Sharon arranged for an interview, and she and I went to meet with the attorney armed with all of Cindy's IEPs from past years. They agreed to take the case.

"Are you ready for a fight? Because it is not going to be easy," the attorney, William, said.

He explained that parents seldom win, mainly because the system is set up so it is too difficult for them to win. Nothing so far in Cindy's life had been easy, so why would we shy away from it now. I assured him I was prepared to do whatever it took. Cindy deserved no less, and she was being wronged. He also explained that in addition to the process being stacked against us, it was also tedious and sometimes boring and I should not expect anything like I see in the movies.

The attorney's first task was to make sure we had as good a hearing officer as possible. The one picked by the school was well known and had a reputation for never ruling in favor of the family.

William was also working on another case with the same hearing officer and managed to successfully object to using him for ours at the same time. So a different hearing officer was assigned. William had no experience with the man but knew he was a school administrator from the area.

PL94-142, The Education for All Handicapped Children Act (1975), stated a definite timeline for due process. According to New York State's regulations, the hearing is supposed to be held and a decision rendered within forty-five days of the initial request, but that timeline was rarely met. We requested the hearing in November 1988, it was held the beginning of February, and the decision made the middle of April. At that time, both parties had the right to appeal the decision to the State Education Department, which had the power to uphold or overturn it. Usually that is as far as things went.

THE HEARING

Although this was just a hearing and held at the school district's offices, it is nonetheless not informal and can be quite intimidating. The school was represented by its attorney, and a court stenographer recorded the entire procedure. A witness list was provided in advance, as well as any evidence. Each side presents their case, and witnesses are sworn in, questioned, and cross-examined just as they are in a courtroom. I remember thinking how awful it must be for a parent who tries to go through this without legal representation. Many families are not able to get free legal help and cannot afford to hire their own, so they go into a hearing with very little support. I can imagine how intimidating it must be to walk into this proceeding with all the "blue suits."

In our hearing one attorney represented the district. The director of special education was also present throughout the hearing, as well as the school principal. On our side was our attorney, William, as well as an educational advocate from his office, Mary, and Bob and me, so we were not outnumbered. Although Sharon was very involved, she was not present but would be called as an expert witness.

The school district called several witnesses, including the director of special education, her assistant director, and the school principal. When testifying, their memory was very good when it came to Cindy's past behaviors. Their testimony was detailed, specific, and very negative. They went into great detail about each outburst.

On cross examination, things were very different.

"Was the teacher for the deaf consulted?"

"I don't recall."

"Was Cindy in a classroom with other students?"

"I don't recall."

"Was Cindy receiving her other services?"

"I don't recall"

"Was Cindy in school?"

"I don't recall."

William told me that was the standard answer to give when the truth would be damaging or a lie. Of course, no one could challenge their memory. Each of their witnesses had excellent memory when it came to anything negative about Cindy, yet each one of them had no recollection of when she was in school. At one point in the hearing, I started to laugh because the response to almost every question posed by William was "I don't recall." The transcript of the hearing, which I requested, had page after page of that same answer from every witness from the district administration.

It seemed as if the school district was trying to give the impression that Cindy had been in a classroom every day all year long, which just was not true. It got to be such an issue that the hearing officer asked to see the attendance records.

The records were brought in the next day, and they actually showed her being in attendance every day. There was, however, a very small asterisk at the bottom of the record, and on the back in small print at the bottom, an explanation that said "as per program." The school's attorney stated the record was proof that Cindy was in school and asked that it be submitted as evidence. William objected as the record was not submitted as evidence in advance as is required. He demanded that if their record was to be admitted, he wanted my calendar showing what days Cindy went to school also to be admitted as evidence. The school's attorney got so upset and got into such a heated discussion that the hearing officer stopped both attorneys and called them into a room across the hall. I assume he told them to calm down and start acting more professionally. Bob and I were amazed that the school district could manipulate records the way they had. William told us that was probably done to get their state aid. Both the school record and mine were admitted as evidence. We were fearful this would hurt our case if the hearing officer believed Cindy was in school every day. That was the major part of our case.

The witnesses for the school district also had very little knowledge about Cindy. Although her IEP stated she should have received the services of a consultant teacher for the deaf, they were unsure if one had been provided. Also, her IEP had a special alert to a behavior management plan, but they could not testify if one was in place. Their testimony was that the intention was to gradually ease Cindy into the classroom. However, there was no formal plan or timeline to do that. Nothing was stated on her individualized educational plan (IEP), which was legally binding.

Also included on the district's witness list was the teacher who originally had Cindy removed from her class. She never testified, and we were convinced it was because they were afraid she would lose her temper and blow it. It would also be difficult for her to say she did not remember if Cindy was in her classroom the last six months or she would have had to lie under oath. Her lack of testimony did not look good for them.

The school district also called Veronica, Cindy's homebound teacher. William was very nervous about her testimony as she was a district employee. He felt strongly she would hurt our case, but I felt differently. I told him I thought she would be honest. It must have been incredibly difficult for her. She confided in me later that she had been getting phone calls from the teacher's union, putting pressure on her about her testimony. Much to her credit, her testimony was honest and forthright and was definitely helpful to our case. Although the district's attorney did not ask, William took a risk and posed the important question.

"Do you think Cindy could be successful in a classroom with other students?" he asked as we held our breath.

"Yes, provided she has the proper supports."

Veronica was also very clear about when Cindy was in school and when she was not. There was not one "I do not recall" response. Testifying as she did, even though she was being truthful, took incredible courage, and she was sure she would never work in the district again. It was a definite plus for our side.

The teaching assistant/interpreter also testified. However, because she lacked credentials, we did not think her testimony made much of an impact. Her testimony consisted mainly of detail about the various incidents. However, upon being cross-examined by our side, it was also obvious her lack of training as an interpreter. The consultant teacher of the deaf was also called to testify. When questioned by our attorney, she stated she had only been involved with Cindy a couple times in the last month. She had never been consulted when Cindy began in the classroom or after the problems began.

Through cross-examination of the school administrators, it was also brought out that there was no behavior management plan, even though the IEP had an alert on it with that reference. They also never consulted with anyone who had prior experience with Cindy.

And they had no formal timeline for what they proposed was a plan to return her to the classroom.

OUR SIDE PRESENTS

Our first witness, Sharon, was wonderful with her testimony. She had done an educational evaluation and written a very favorable report. She had all the necessary credentials and made a very credible witness. And she had known Cindy for years and observed her in several different settings. Her testimony was very helpful to our side of course, and she also did well on the cross-examination.

Our witnesses also included an independent psychologist who had tested Cindy. We had hired this person as he had experience testing individuals with disabilities. I did not trust the school district psychologist to do her testing. A special education teacher who had worked with Cindy over the summer also testified, as did the director of her summer program through the Association for the Hearing Impaired. Except for the psychologist, all our witnesses had long-term relationships with Cindy. And they all came with excellent credentials.

Before the hearing we hired a consultant who specialized in deaf education to give us an independent evaluation. She came highly recommended and she understood she would be testifying at the hearing. She was supposed to have everything done by the end of December but she did not. She spoke with Sharon and she visited the school. Her report arrived in February, two days before the hearing. Fortunately, because we were paying her bill, it came directly to us. I could not believe my eyes when I read it.

The report was based on two visits: one to school where she spent the time in a staff meeting and the other to Cindy's job site. She never spoke to us or anyone at St. Mary's. Her only input came from the school, and she never observed Cindy with her homebound teacher or even spoke directly with that teacher. She began her report with a background saying that Cindy came from a residential school for the deaf and was put into a regular classroom of typical hearing students with no preparation at all. Later in her report, she wrote how harmful the effects were of dumping special education students into regular classes without proper support. The entire rest of the report was based on that premise. I immediately called her and asked if she was aware that Cindy was never in a "regular" classroom but was in a self-contained special education classroom with a special education teacher and an interpreter and there was considerable preparation. She admitted she did not know any of that. She had no clue what had happened and was totally under the wrong impression. I gave her some background, which she should have asked for long before, and requested she reconsider her report. She told me she would do that and send me a revised report.

The only change in the revised report was that she changed the word "regular" classroom to "special education" classroom. I could not believe it and neither could our attorney. She based her entire report on a false premise and then merely changed a couple of words, totally changing that original premise. We all agreed that the report would be damaging. I called her and told her that under no circumstances was she to release that report to anyone without my permission. She told me that the school district had contacted her and said they could call her as a witness and if called she would have to testify. I reminded her of her requirement of confidentiality and told her in no uncertain terms was she to violate it. Because her name had been on our witness list, the school district was questioning why she was not testifying, and they were pushing the issue. It was obvious they knew the report was not favorable and were trying hard to get it admitted. But, thank God because we were paying the bill, it was up to us to release it and of course we refused. The hearing officer questioned the existence of the evaluation and who paid for it. When told it was paid for by us, the matter was dropped. The consultant was never called as a witness, but just the fact that she did not testify hurt our case as it was assumed her report would not have helped us. It was not looking good for us.

OUR LAST-MINUTE WITNESS RUSHES IN AND OUT

In addition, I had been trying to reach Martha, the behavior consultant at St. Mary's, but she had not returned my phone calls. The evening of the second day of the hearing, she called and asked if we still needed her. I managed to get a message to our attorney, and he said yes by all means. So, the plan was that she would fly in the next morning to testify. Bob would leave the hearing to pick her up at the airport and bring her back to the hearing, as it was expected it would wrap up in the morning. During testimony in the morning, someone came in and handed me a note saying Martha's flight had been delayed by weather; she would not be arriving until noon or so. William explained to the others and asked that we adjourn for lunch early and reconvene so the witness could be heard. All agreed and Bob, William, and I went to the airport to get Martha. Her plane was late of course, and when she arrived, I asked William to let me greet her first. We hugged and I told her how very grateful we were for her coming.

We rode directly back to the hearing and on the way William prepared Martha for her testimony. She gave a wonderful testimony, which was very favorable to us. She stressed the importance of a behavior management plan and the need for someone with training in working with the deaf. She spoke about Cindy's behaviors being a form of communication. Immediately after her testimony, she left with Bob for the airport to catch a flight back. We adjourned only long enough for me to say goodbye and thank you. It was truly something right out of a Perry Mason movie, with the last-minute witness being rushed into the court and rushed right back out. William had told me in the beginning not to expect any big drama, but this seemed like good material for a John Grisham novel. Score another point for our side.

The hearing lasted three days and was incredibly tense and draining, with many highs and lows. We would suffer through a bad blow and then be picked up by an incredible score. It was an emotional roller-coaster. Contrary to what William had told us, this was definitely not boring. I had wanted William to call me as a witness, and I think he was close to doing it. But when all the tension and drama happened with Martha and the delays, I became very nervous. I think he was afraid to take the chance. I hoped he was right. William was positively incredible and absolutely a relentless cross-examiner. He never backed down for one minute and never missed a trick. I sat close to him, and anytime someone gave wrong information or left out something, I would pass a note to him and he would follow up. He is a man of small stature with a huge presence during proceedings. He definitely outdid the district's attorney.

THE DECISION

The decision came a little more than thirty days after the hearing and was more than we expected. Not only did the officer rule in our favor and put Cindy back in a classroom, but he also mandated a full-time teacher for the deaf. The hearing officer also stated in his decision that the question of whether or not Cindy was in school was still unclear, but he suspected my records were truthful. Apparently, he was more in tune with what had been going on than we thought and was truly being fair in the process. This was a huge win for us, and we were thrilled. But the battle was far from over. William told us to expect the district to appeal the decision, and within a few days, we were served with yet another summons. It was something to which we would become accustomed. Whenever a stranger appeared at the door and asked for us, we instantly knew they were there to serve us papers.

Cheryl Kantak

STILL NO CLASSROOM FOR CINDY

There was a question of whether the school had to abide by the decision while the appeal process took place, and we felt that they did. However, the school did not agree with that, and they did not return Cindy to the classroom. There was a required timeline for the appeal process, so William was busy preparing his briefs in response to the district's petition to appeal. They had to be in Albany by a required date. If they were not, the decision would automatically be overturned. Cindy had still not been returned to the classroom.

In June, Cindy had a difficult morning at her job site. Although she was fine later that day when she returned to school, as well as the next day, the following day she was suspended from school for the remainder of the year. Because of the way it had been handled, we filed a discrimination suit with the Office of Civil Rights (OCR). It had been the second time we had filed with them. Shortly after this all began, we filed a complaint that Cindy was being discriminated against with the interpreter. She was not a qualified interpreter and was being paid as a teaching assistant. Elsewhere in the district, there was another student who functioned much higher than Cindy receiving the services of a certified interpreter who was paid at that level. OCR ruled against us in both those complaints. There were so many suits being filed from both sides, it was difficult for a lay person to keep it all straight.

WE WIN AGAIN BUT STILL NO CLASSROOM

In September 1989, the State Education Department upheld the original hearing officer's decision completely and further ordered the district to put Cindy back into the classroom with a full-time teacher for the deaf. It was another huge win for us, and we thought we were home free. Of course, the district had the right to take it to the next step and appeal that decision and that is exactly what they did.

First, the school district filed a petition to the Commissioner to reopen the decision. Our attorney had to file a response, which he told us was submitted on time. It was delivered in the evening of the last day. Shortly after, our attorney received a letter from the State Education Department saying the papers were not filed on time and the decision would be overturned. Failure to respond means you concede and lose. It turned out to be confusion on the part of the State Education Department. A security guard let the delivery person in the building, and the papers were left on a conference room table where they were discovered days later. Proof of delivery was provided; the delay of the papers was the fault of the state and the case was back in process. It was just one more piece of nerve-racking tension. And we were told there would be no drama? In February 1990, the Commissioner denied the district's motion to reopen on the basis of time and merit.

Next, the district filed suit in State Supreme Court to have the Commissioner's decision set aside. It was not too long before we were once again being served papers. It was hard to believe, but the district was not going to let this go. Many people who were knowledgeable about what was going on could not believe they were continuing to fight this. I think it had become personal with the superintendent who did not like to lose and did not want to set a precedent. If he had to provide a teacher for the deaf for one student, he was most likely afraid that there would be more knocking at his door trying to return to their home schools.

WE GO TO FEDERAL COURT

Even though the state had ordered the school district to put Cindy back into a classroom and provide a full-time teacher for the deaf, they still did not do so. They continued to maintain they did not have to abide by the decision until the appeals process was complete. In September 1989, Cindy returned to school in a special education class but without the teacher for the deaf. She had already lost an entire school year. Now this school year was half over, and Cindy still was not getting what she was supposed to be getting. We were all furious and could not believe they were violating the orders of the State Education Department. The district maintained that as long as there was an appeal in process, they did not have to abide by the ruling. The district had now filed suit with the NYS Supreme Court to have the Commissioner's decision set aside. This could take years and William was not about to wait. He decided to go to Federal Court to seek an injunction. That would be something that could not be ignored. He also submitted a motion to have the State Supreme Court case moved to the Federal Court. He initiated the process, and when the case was heard, I went to Federal Court to observe. It was all very impressive to me, and he presented his case beautifully. Once again, we had to wait for the judge's decision.

BEING IN THE PUBLIC EYE IS NO FUN

While we were waiting, William thought it might be good to get a little publicity, and he contacted the local newspaper. A reporter came to our house and wrote a story about our fight with the district. We were featured on the front page of the local section. The article gave the details of the lawsuit over Cindy's program as well as describing her disabilities. It also mentioned we had another daughter with disabilities who was in an inclusive program in the district. At the time the article was written, we were still awaiting the decision from Federal Court. I wasn't sure when the article was going to appear but found out when I received an unexpected call early one Sunday morning from a total stranger. He told me he was thrilled I was trying to get the district to do the right thing because he had tried also but had been unsuccessful. He was very kind and encouraging and wished us luck.

A short while later, I received another phone call from a not-so-nice woman. She was outraged and said some horrible things to me. I was so taken aback and surprised by it that I started to defend myself. Bob was standing close by and realized what was happening and was trying to get me to hang up. This woman told me I was irresponsible for bringing two "defective" children into the world and how dare I expect her to pay to educate them. She told me I should keep them home where they belong and not expect the school district to deal with them. She also asked why I didn't have an amniocentesis. I tried to explain to her that I did have that but it was a very limited test and would only show certain things and would not show my daughter's disabilities. I tried to tell her she did not know what she was talking about but she kept screaming terrible things at me until I finally hung up in tears. I could not believe the cruelty of this person. Now, I wonder if that call was from someone indirectly involved in the case purposefully trying to intimidate us or if it was truly a random call.

Unfortunately, that phone call was not the last one like it. That afternoon someone called wanting to know if we lived near a landfill or major power lines and if we knew the cause of our daughters' problems. It seemed like every nut-case in the area had a theory or opinion about our girls. It was horrible, and finally we stopped answering the phone. The next day we purchased an answering machine so we could screen the calls. Being the center of media attention is no fun.

It was fortunate we had the answering machine, because the judge's decision came the following morning. He ruled in our favor and granted us the injunction. This time the story made the headlines of the front page, and our phone was ringing constantly. The television stations were now airing the story, and reporters kept calling for comments. The school district superintendent was interviewed on camera and asked point blank if he would ignore the injunction. He replied that he could not do that and would follow the judge's order. He also said they would decide whether they would appeal the decision.

So, with less than two weeks left in the school year, Cindy would finally get her full-time teacher for the deaf. It had taken two full school years. Of course, because of the timing, getting anything in place wasn't worth it for a few days. But come September, Cindy would start school in a classroom with the proper supports.

All during this process, we had continually told Cindy that we were working to get her back in the class. Though we tried our best to explain what was going on, there was no way she could comprehend the complexity of the situation. But she knew and sensed our reactions through all of it. I know she understood our anger and tension, and when the decisions from the hearing and court proceeding came in, she shared our joy and excitement. It was difficult for her when she didn't go back to the classroom right away, and we had a difficult time making her understand it. We ourselves could not understand how the district was able to ignore the rulings. If the decision had not been in our favor, then we would have had no choice but to abide by it, but they choose to ignore it. In the newspaper article, I was quoted as saying we had gone through the system and played by the rules, and yet the school district totally ignored the rules. The article was not particularly favorable to the school district.

THE DISTRICT IS STILL FIGHTING US

Although Cindy would now be getting everything that had been ordered, the district was continuing the appeals process. Lawsuits were being filed by the school district against the Commissioner of Education in State Supreme Court but were moved to Federal Court. Shortly after the injunction was granted, the district also filed suit in the U.S. 2nd Circuit Court. Once the appeals process reached the 2nd Circuit Court, William explained that it is handled differently.

Briefs are submitted by both sides as always, but they are given to a committee of the court. The purpose of this committee is to try to resolve the cases before they are actually heard and lessen the court's caseload. Members of the committee review the briefs and speak with the attorneys. We never knew what was said to the school district's attorney, but eventually the district dropped the case. We never knew if they were told they had no case or if the district just finally gave up. Also, the federal judge eventually ruled against the district in its appeal to set aside the decision. It was finally over. It had gone as far as it could go. Because we prevailed, the school district was now responsible for all the costs involved, including our attorney. Even though we did not have to pay him, he could now sue the district for his fees and did just that.

It was almost six years after all this mess started that the two parties settled. One day, I received in the mail two checks totaling $20,000. This was the amount that both sides settled on for our attorney fees. While it may not have been much to the school district, it would have been monumental to us if we had to pay it. The school district also had to pay all the hearing costs as well as their attorney fees. The checks were made out to me because I am Cindy's parent and legal guardian. Boy did it feel good to get that money, even though I knew it wasn't mine. I joked about cashing the check and letting them come after me for the money but of course I didn't do that. It was a fitting end to a long and painful fight.

The truly ironic thing about the whole affair is that the teacher who initiated all these difficulties left her class and became a resource teacher. I never knew if it was a voluntary transfer or not. Her replacement was none other than Veronica, and she was hired by the same director of special education that testified against us. It reinforced our feeling that she was on our side all along but was being told what to do by her superior. I suppose I cannot fault her for that as I am sure she valued her job, but it stunk nonetheless. It was wonderful that she recognized the talent and credibility of

Veronica and turned around and hired her. She was one of Cindy's teachers for the remainder of her time at the high school and was also Deb's teacher when she was in high school. Cindy had a couple of different teachers for the deaf, but Veronica remained a constant and really became a friend to our family. She was, and I suspect still is, a wonderful teacher and person, and it is rare to find someone like her.

CINDY MADE HER MARK

Several years after the hearing, I co-presented at a conference in New Orleans. The Center on Human Policy at Syracuse University had sent me and two other women to do a workshop about residential services. One of them I knew well but I had just met the other. We were out on the town one night walking down Bourbon Street and getting to know each other. Kathy had asked me about my children, and I mentioned that we had a major battle with our school district. She asked me for more details, and when I gave them to her, she suddenly stopped walking and said, "That was you?" She explained she had attended a conference the previous year in California and in one of the workshops heard about this case. No names were used so she didn't know who it was at the time but it was definitely Cindy. It had been used as an example of legal action that could be taken.

A short while later, a friend of mine sent me a copy of a page from a law review and right there in black and white was our case. Going to Federal Court to seek an injunction had set legal precedent, and Cindy had made her mark once again. She also paved the way for other students who are deaf to return to their local district, and a few years after the hearing, I received a call from a parent trying to do just that. Cindy helped that family.

Silent Crusader

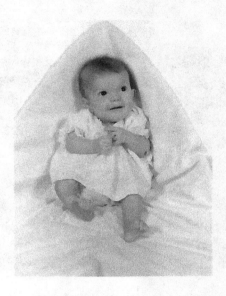

Cindy 7 months old before leg surgeries

Cheryl Kantak

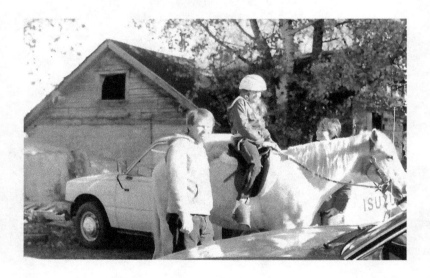

Cindy and Dad. She loves horses

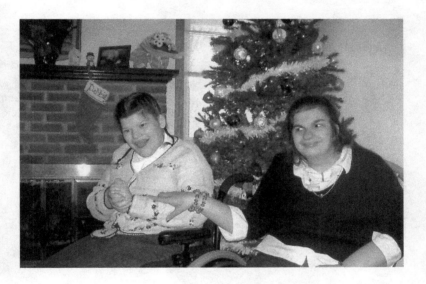

Deb and Cindy at Deb's house

Cheryl Kantak

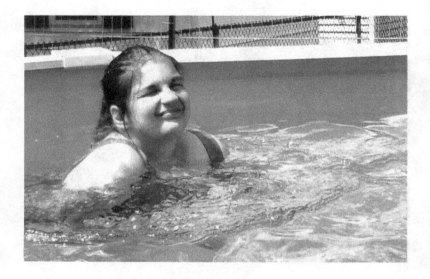

Cindy swims like a fish

Silent Crusader

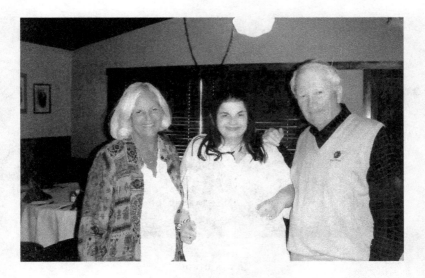

Cindy's 40th birthday

Cheryl Kantak

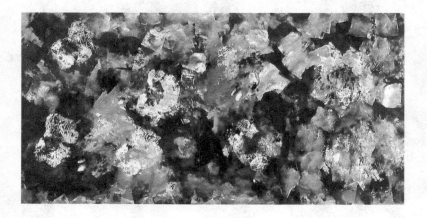

Cindy's artwork

Silent Crusader

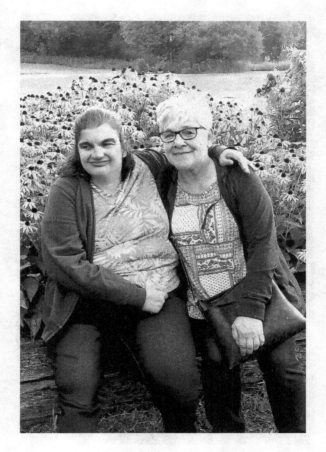

Cindy and Cheryl twelve years together

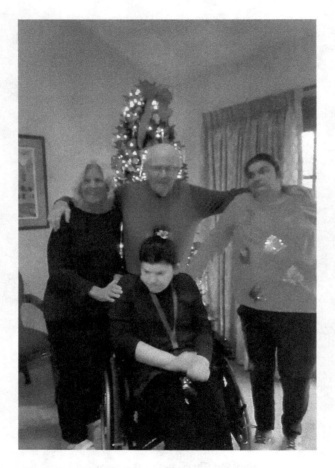

Our family

Chapter 7
THE FIGHT TOOK ITS TOLL; CINDY MOVES OUT

After Cindy returned to school to Veronica's class with her full-time teacher for the deaf, things were much better, although there were still problems. Cindy by this time was exhibiting some challenging behaviors both at home and in school. We had started to see some grabbing and throwing things at the tail end of her time at St. Mary's, but it had been getting progressively worse. It was very difficult for Cindy to get up at 5:00 a.m. so that she could get the bus at 7:00. She did not sleep well at night and was a bear to awaken. It would not be unusual for her to grab me or throw something. She could be sitting at the kitchen table having her breakfast and suddenly throw her orange juice or even flip over the entire table. Some of these behaviors were also seen in school, but fortunately, Veronica dealt with them. Cindy would rip things, including pictures and important papers, and frequently threw her hearing aids. One time when replacing her hearing aids, the dealer told me they probably were not of much use to her anyway. Over time, she wore them less and less and finally not at all.

Cindy became more and more aggressive, and eventually this took its toll on all of us, including Debbie. One time Cindy threw a framed picture at our front window near where Deb was playing on the floor. The glass in the frame shattered, and Deb started screaming. Deb was not hurt, but she startles easily and does not like loud noises. It took a long time to calm Deb down. We would sometimes be able to tell when this was going to happen and would take precautions of removing objects from Cindy's reach. But other times there would be no warning, and it would seem to come out of the blue. It became very difficult to live that way, and we were all suffering. Her sign language skills are limited, and we felt her behavior was a form of communication. We knew Cindy was unhappy but we didn't know how to help her.

NO REST FOR THE WEARY

It was also very difficult for Bob and me to get away from it. When you have two children with disabilities, respite is extremely hard to get. Going out for just a few hours becomes a monumental task requiring weeks of preparation. We were hooked up with all the local agencies and services, but finding people to provide the respite was terribly hard. At one point Bob and I hired people at our expense to take the girls out into the community and do things with them so we could have some time. We advertised and interviewed and found some terrific people for each of the girls. One woman who applied for the job with Cindy was an attorney who worked in the same office that handled our case with the school district. Although she was applying for the job with Cindy, we felt she was a better match for Deb and asked her if she would be interested in working with her. She did that for several years until she moved out of state. Each of the girls had their own special friend and their own activities. Unfortunately, they didn't always go out at the same time, but we did get some of the break that we so desperately needed.

One time we had arranged through an agency for someone to stay with the girls for an evening so we could go to a special dinner dance. We met with the person a couple of times and filled her in about both the girls, including Cindy's behaviors. She assured us she had lots of experience and would have no problems handling Cindy. I hoped so because this was a formal affair, and Bob and I were both looking forward to it. It was not something we did often, and I had a new dress and went all out for the big occasion. The dinner was held at a local hotel, and there were several hundred people in attendance. We had cocktails before dinner and had been seated just a short time at the dinner table. Soon a waiter came to our table looking for us to let us know there was a phone call. We were seated toward the front of the room, and a good friend had just taken the stage to begin the program of festivities. When I took the call, our sitter was in tears saying she could not deal with Cindy. Cindy was grabbing and throwing things and would we please come home immediately. I stood at the door of the dining room and saw Bob was looking my way. I only had to motion to him to come, and he picked up everything, knowing we were headed home. We never got to eat the dinner. After the sitter left, Cindy was just fine.

There would be many more times like that where our plans were changed or canceled because of Cindy's behavior. There were daily struggles with Cindy, and she was the focus of most of our attention. Deb was so placid but seemed to keep her distance from Cindy. She clearly did not like it when Cindy acted out. Deb prefers a calm, quiet atmosphere. Cindy, on the other hand, often makes quick sudden moves and tends to slam doors, not realizing it is offensive to others. The girls get along for the most part, and I believe they love each other. But they have their own very different personalities and temperaments.

A LITTLE RESPITE FOR US

Arranging for time away was very difficult. But occasionally, we did manage to arrange for the girls to spend some time in respite. A couple of times, they went to a state-run group home about thirty miles away that was nicknamed the "country club." It was a large beautiful house on a lake that had about a dozen people living there. It was called an intermediate care facility (ICF). Because of the high level of need and medical issues of the people living there, it had more staff. Neither Cindy nor Deb did very well there. Cindy clearly did not like being in a group of people with such intense needs. Deb was so easy going that they paid little attention to her.

Cindy also spent some time in other group homes and, for the most part, was not happy in any of them. Cindy did not like to have to conform to the ways of others. There was one house for four women where she spent several weekends. It was the best of all the ones she had been to but she still had problems. Because one of the women had to go to the hospital early every Saturday morning for blood tests, everyone had to get out of bed and go with her because there was only one staff. Cindy clearly did not like that. Also, even though Cindy had always slept with the door of her bedroom open, she was required to keep it closed. That was the nature of a group home and all the rules that go along with them, and Cindy was not happy in them. Perhaps they reminded her of the rigidity of St. Mary's, and she resented the loss of her freedom.

Cindy did the best in houses where the people functioned on a higher level. I think that was because Cindy does not consider herself to be disabled and does not like being grouped with people with disabilities. It is interesting because that is common for deaf people. Many deaf people do not consider themselves to have a disability, and someone like Cindy who obviously has other issues besides her hearing loss is not always accepted by the deaf community. She is somewhat caught between two worlds, not really a part of either. People sometimes have a hard time believing that until they actually witness the rejection.

SEEKING HELP FROM DOCTORS

At one point Cindy's behavior became so difficult that on the advice of her internist we sought the help of a psychiatrist. We were referred to one that worked in the clinic at the District Service Office of the Office of Mental Retardation and Developmental Disabilities (OMRDD). I had been consulting with Sarah, my case worker from that same office. She accompanied me and Cindy to the appointment where we discussed medication. In addition to her behaviors, Cindy was also wetting the bed at night.

The doctor decided to start her on Tofranil and began with a very low dose. We saw results almost immediately, with Cindy seeming calmer and no wet beds. We were thrilled and returned for the follow-up a few weeks later with the good report. The doctor was pleased but said she was not at therapeutic level and he was going to double the dosage. I questioned whether that was necessary seeing she was doing so well, but he insisted despite my concerns.

Shortly after the dosage was increased, Cindy did not appear to be as calm as she had been. She was not acting right and was showing more signs of frustration. It is so difficult to try and figure out what is going on with her sometimes, and she just is not able to tell us. I became concerned that perhaps she was not feeling well and took her to her internist. When the doctor took her blood pressure, she told me she wanted the Tofranil stopped immediately and she would call the psychiatrist and speak to him. Apparently, it had caused her blood pressure to skyrocket. She was so concerned that she asked me to get a blood pressure kit and monitor it for the next week and call her if it didn't start coming down. Cindy improved dramatically in the next couple of days, and her blood pressure returned to normal. I was so angry at the psychiatrist for insisting on the increase in the dosage and furious at myself for letting him. We never went back to him, and I became very leery of giving Cindy any medicine that was not necessary.

The bedwetting had started gradually in her last year at St. Mary's and had continued after she came home. I had consulted with her pediatrician at the time and was told not to make a big deal of it. I followed his advice and just continued to wash the sheets. I was afraid if I had her wear something, she would perceive it as permission. Eventually it became an everyday occurrence. Cindy was always very nervous any time her doctor tried to examine her lower abdomen, and she would always pull on her underwear to protect herself. Her doctor never pushed it and told me that people with disabilities sometimes felt violated by such an exam.

When she was old enough and I switched her to an internist, I once again addressed the issue of bedwetting. Despite the wonderful rapport between Cindy and her internist, she still did not get a thorough examination and she decided to send her to a specialist. That specialist, a male, was not very sympathetic or understanding of Cindy's disabilities. When I explained how protective and nervous she was, he defiantly told me he had examined very young children and he would get an exam whether she cooperated or not. I told him it was a very real possibility he could get his glasses ripped off his face but he was not impressed. We decided he would order some tests first. Two different tests would be done. They required that an IV be inserted and then a solution injected and X-rays taken. Cindy would have to hold her urine and then release it on request. I told him I was not sure we would be able to get that kind of understanding or cooperation from her, but we would try.

When the time came, Cindy had to go through the ordeal of cleansing her bowels, and despite the unpleasantness, she was cooperative. When we went for the tests at a radiologist's office close to our home, Cindy was very nervous. Although she was cooperative, her anxiousness was obvious. A doctor came to start an IV, and Cindy willingly gave him her arm. With me by her side as always, trying to comfort and soothe her, he tried to get a line started. His first few attempts failed, and he tried the other arm. He was having an awful time because Cindy's veins are deep and sometimes difficult to hit. The doctor was sweating terribly and was noticeably uncomfortable with the situation. At one time, he left the room and came back to try again. After about twenty minutes, he declared failure and said she would have to have it done in the hospital where they had phlebotomists. I could not put Cindy through all that again. Every time Cindy had to go through something like that, we worried she would regress back to the times when she would scream through every appointment.

My fear of traumatizing her had kept me from doing things I should have done. Although she had seen a gynecologist, she had never had an internal exam for that very reason. Cindy has also never had a menstrual cycle, something I have always considered to be truly a gift. I do not know how she would handle it and I have always been thankful I have never had to find out. She did have a sonogram, and it showed she has a uterus although it is very small. I had been getting pressure from both doctors and state personnel to get her an exam and realized that my reluctance and fears were not helping her. I knew I had to deal with it. I could have easily had someone else take her and totally avoid participating in it but I felt that doing so would be abandoning her. I have seen her through everything and felt a need to see her through this. It took me several years, but I finally found a wonderful caring gynecologist who did her initial exam in the one-day surgery center while Cindy was sedated. She continues to follow both girls.

THE PROBLEMS AT SCHOOL CONTINUE

Although Veronica was a terrific teacher and Cindy did well with her, there were still problems in school. The program was community-based, and the class would learn skills while making trips to the mall, banks, laundromats, and the like. Also, the students went to various job sites where they had specific goals and earned a very small amount for achieving them — a dollar per goal per day. They would receive a "paycheck" and then deposit it in the bank. The woman who did the job-matching, Peggy B., and I did not see eye to eye when it came to Cindy or much else for that matter. While she was required to match Cindy with a job, she was very vocal about her opinion that the best place for Cindy would be a sheltered workshop. When I told her I felt that would be the worst place to put Cindy and it would only happen over my dead body, our problems began. I had visited the workshops and explained that Cindy did not like segregated settings or repetitive work. I felt she would become bored very quickly and would not like the setting. As a result, she would end up acting out, which would eventually lead to her being removed from the program. Putting her in a sheltered workshop would set her up for failure.

It was difficult at times to find the right job match for Cindy, as sometimes her behaviors interfered and workers did not always tolerate them well. But instead of trying to work through the difficulties or trying harder to find a better match, Cindy was just removed from the job site. She spent some time working in a restaurant cleaning tables and setting tables. She worked at a hotel doing some cleaning of rooms where one of the employees was very supportive of her. She worked in an office of a local agency that served people with disabilities, and surprisingly, the people there were not particularly tolerant of Cindy's inappropriate behaviors. Other job sites included a day care center, a home for the elderly, a manufacturer where she packed pencils into a box, and the laundry room of a hotel.

When the deaf education consultant made her visit during our hearing with the district, she saw Cindy at work in the laundry folding towels. One of the few positive remarks in her report was that a better effort should be made to help Cindy understand her job. Her example was that a large bin of cleans towels came to Cindy from another place in the hotel. She was expected to fold the towels and put them on a shelf. From her viewpoint, they would remain there until someone came in and took them. Then she would get another bin of unfolded towels. No one ever explained to her why she was doing the folding or where they came from or went. So, she was finally given a tour where dirty towels were removed from a room, taken to the laundry, and eventually put in the bin. They were then brought to her room for folding and stacking and then removed and put in a freshly cleaned room. It was such an easy thing to do and helped Cindy understand the whole picture.

Whenever there were any problems on the job site, a meeting would be called and I was always asked to offer some solutions. I often did that, but it was difficult because parents were not allowed to visit the job site. In fact, even if Cindy needed to be picked up early for an appointment, parents were still not allowed at the job site. The reason given for this was because it was a place of employment, but the rule angered me and other parents as well. I felt I might be able to offer some help if I had been allowed to try. One time I just plain refused to abide by the stupid rule because doing so would have taken me way out of my way for nothing. I needed to pick up Cindy for a doctor's appointment. I was close to her job site, which was also close to the doctor's office. It was ridiculous for me to drive all the way back to the high school only to drive her back to only a few blocks from her job. So I wrote a note to Veronica and told her I would be picking Cindy up at her job site. It was incredibly simple and there were no problems, but it irritated Peggy.

To make matters worse, Peggy seldom consulted with the teachers involved with the students, despite their offers of help. Peggy had her own staff of job coaches who were given a set of goals for the students. The job coaches rotated between several students but rarely had any contact with parents or even the teaching staff. Eventually, Cindy ended up with a so-called job in the school cafeteria because Peggy said that there would be no one in the community that would hire her. While I admit that Cindy was not an enthusiastic employee and that competitive employment would be difficult, the attitude and preconceived ideas of this woman irritated me to no end, and I never hesitated to tell her. I also occasionally took the opportunity to irritate her as much as she did me. After Cindy left high school, Peggy got divorced. She not only went back to her maiden name but also started going by Margaret instead of Peggy. Shortly after Deb entered high school, I received a letter from a Margaret S. I wasn't sure who it was. Veronica, who was then Deb's teacher, informed me Peggy had divorced and went back to her maiden name. She also told people she had always hated the name Peggy. She was formally using Margaret now and wanted others to do the same. One time during a meeting, she was being extremely negative about Deb and her future. She had not changed at all from when Cindy was in school, and I was becoming more irritated as she continued to speak. So I made a point to call her Peggy, corrected myself once and then continued using Peggy. She knew I was purposely doing it to irritate her and so did everyone else. I think Veronica had a hard time holding back her smile.

TIME FOR CINDY TO MOVE OUT

As Cindy approached her late teens, and Bob and I became more tired, we began to think about Cindy living somewhere else. Cindy did not seem happy at home any longer, and life was very difficult for us. As a result of my involvement in committees and boards, and my job with the Parent Training Project, I was knowledgeable about the residential system and how it worked. I was also on the board of directors of a local agency serving people with disabilities and was up to date on what was happening with the development of group homes.

The agency was a private not-for-profit (NFP) agency located in central New York that provided a variety of services to people with disabilities. Started primarily by a group of parents and concerned citizens, they were committed to provide better service in smaller settings. Initially, they opened three six-person group homes, which was virtually unheard of at the time. I knew that the waiting list in our county was very long, and people waited many years before being placed in a group home. When an opening did come up, it wasn't always something a parent wanted, but many felt they had to take it or wait years more. The state system of residential placement is not especially user-friendly. I had also been part of a citizen review committee that evaluated group homes, and of course, my daughters had done respite at several of them.

While on the board, I was the chair of their selection committee, which was responsible for choosing the residents for the new group homes they opened. I participated in that selection process for two of their homes. Knowing what I knew about group homes, I had decided that I was going to make the selections the right way and not just throw people together. I put together a committee of very talented people, and we began the tedious task of looking at names on the waiting list. At that time, private not-for-profit agencies were required to fill half the beds in any house they opened with people from the State Developmental Center. The state was trying to move people out of the institutions so they could eventually close them, something many people had advocated for. The funding for new group homes, or community residences as they are called, was linked to the closure of the institution, and taking people from the institution was a condition of receiving funding.

We met on a regular basis, and I took the task very seriously, as did the others. We reviewed and talked about each person and slowly narrowed down the possibilities. We then split into teams and visited everyone. It was a horrendous job, and I felt a little like I was playing God. It was so hard saying no to some of the families. Our committee put in a great deal of time and effort, and we thought we had done a good job of matching people.

Because I was on the board of the agency, I was able to see and hear firsthand how the house worked once folks moved in. I was terribly upset when I watched things start to fall apart because the people who lived at the house did not get along at all. Two of the women we purposely chose because they knew each other before and had roomed together in the past. What we found out later was they disliked one another and did poorly together. They were both nonverbal and could not tell us. Unfortunately, their files never gave any indication of their previous relationship, and the people who knew them and had the opportunity to tell us never did so. They had a long history, which people chose not to give us, probably because they just wanted to see them move out of the institution. There were many other problems at the house, and one person was removed by their family. Years later, the people living in that home decided to live in even smaller homes or their own home. The house was sold to another agency.

What I learned from that experience is that no matter how hard you try, you just cannot match people. If you are going to throw six or eight or more people together in one living arrangement, you are going to have problems. It is not always a bad situation, and in fact, the second house where I helped select the residents worked well for many years. I am not saying all group homes are bad, just that I personally do not like the concept. I strongly believe that individuals/families should have options so they can choose a setting they feel is the best suited for their loved one.

What I also knew is that Cindy did not like group homes much better than I did, which left Bob and me with a huge dilemma. Group homes of one type or another were the only choice we had, and even getting into one of those was extremely difficult. The waiting list was very long, and openings rarely came up.

OUR IDEA

We talked a great deal about the options or lack of them and began to think about doing something different. We knew we would not be paying for a college education for either girl, and a big formal wedding was probably not going to happen either. So we came up with the idea of buying the girls a house of their own. We thought that Cindy could live there now, and Deb could respite there occasionally. When it came time for Deb to move out, she would also have a place to live. It would be a huge financial commitment for us, but compared to the cost of college and formal weddings, it really wasn't that bad. The problem, of course, and the biggest cost, would be the staffing, and that was something we could not afford.

We started talking with agencies and people at the District Service Office (DSO), the local office of the state's OMRDD (Office of Mental Retardation and Developmental Disabilities). We found this was a fairly novel idea. At the time, the late '80s, there were only one or two other similar arrangements in the entire state that we knew about.

We finally got to talk with an administrative person at our local OMRDD office and proposed to him that we would take responsibility for the house and related costs if the state would find a way to staff it. It took a very long time and many meetings to get an answer, but finally we were told that if we purchased the house, the state would certify it as a family care home and look for a family care provider to live there with Cindy. By this time, I had become very involved with the local not-for-profit (NFP) agency and felt strongly about its philosophy that smaller settings were better. When I asked the state people if that agency could oversee the house, I was told no because they were not currently certified to do family care. The only way we could do this was with the state overseeing the house. We really had no choice but to go along with it and proceeded to find a house. We purposely looked for a ranch-style house for accessibility for Deb. It also had to be in the same school district, because Cindy was still in school and I did not want to switch districts and have to fight all over again for services.

Cheryl Kantak

OUR FIRST PROVIDER — NOT A GREAT FIRST IMPRESSION

It took us a while to find the house, and by the time we did, the state had identified a potential family care provider. I had met her before when I was asked to moderate a rally that was held when the state tried to cut family care funding. The DSO provided a sitter so I could attend the rally. Ann Marie came to the house and met me and both the girls. She was to come early in the morning and finish getting Deb off to school and then leave. Cindy would have already left by the time she arrived. It was only for a short time, and I had as much done for her as possible. I specifically told her that when she left to please make sure the front door was pulled tightly closed and check to make sure it locked. I explained we were having a problem with it, and if it wasn't closed tightly, the wind would blow it open. She assured me she would make sure it was closed and locked.

The rally was a huge success, and I did not return home until almost 2:00 that afternoon. When I arrived, I found the front door to my house was wide open. I was furious and called the person who had set up the arrangement. She contacted Ann Marie, who then called me to tell me that indeed she pulled hard to shut the door and checked that it was locked. There wasn't anything I could do about it, but I wanted her to know that the door was wide open when I got home. I thanked her for her time, wished her luck, and our conversation ended on a friendly note. It was months later when my case worker at the state told me that the potential family care provider was Ann Marie. I was surprised, and my immediate reaction was not positive but I was encouraged to keep an open mind. I was told, "Family care providers are hard to find."

Ann Marie was a junior at Syracuse University, majoring in special education. The state was encouraging me to accept her as the family care provider. She came to visit again, and we talked and she interviewed well. She wanted to know if she could also ask a close friend to move into the house so they could share some of the responsibility. I expressed concern to my case worker about a second person but was reminded how difficult it was to find people willing to do this. Bob and I were just plain exhausted and craved some relief.

We met with Ann Marie and her friend several times. We had some concerns about the friend because of the questions she was asking. Instead of wanting details about Cindy, she was the most concerned about whether there would be a TV in the house and if she could bring her lounge chair with the heat massage. When I expressed my concerns to the folks at the state, I was reminded that the friend was not the family care provider, and we should be as accommodating as we can to Ann Marie because "providers are hard to find." So, with some reservations mixed with our eagerness to make the change, we agreed to move forward.

CINDY MOVES INTO HER HOME

Late in September 1991, at the age of nineteen, Cindy moved into her own home. Cindy was very excited about the move and so were we. We visited the house beforehand and furnished it with some things Cindy was familiar with. We also shopped together and bought her many new furnishings. It was very exciting for all of us. We felt confident that this move was what Cindy wanted. Bob and I were looking forward to a somewhat easier time and the prospect of some time for ourselves. We hoped having only Deb with us would ease the task of finding childcare and we would be able to get out more often. It was also our hope that Deb could spend some time at Cindy's on occasion so Bob and I could have a weekend alone. It seemed like the perfect solution for everyone.

We made every attempt we could to make sure Ann Marie and her friend were comfortable and felt supported. We gave Ann Marie the largest bedroom with the private bath. Cindy took the smallest bedroom. Ann Marie's friend took the second largest bedroom, which had a nice closet. She and Cindy would share the second bathroom. Everyone agreed to the arrangements and appeared happy with them. We had close contact with the girls those first few weeks, and things seemed to be going along nicely.

A few weeks after Cindy moved into her home, Bob and I were out celebrating our anniversary. Obtaining childcare for only Deb was a little easier. Bob and I were sitting having our dinner, reflecting on how wonderful it was to be able to go out without having to worry about being called back, when the waiter came over and told us we had a phone call. It was our sitter telling us to call Cindy's house immediately. Cindy had been acting out, and the roommate was upset and called our house trying to get in touch with us. We left without finishing our meal and went directly to Cindy's.

When we arrived, Ann Marie was on the phone with the emergency contact person at the state. Cindy had started to throw things and grab at the girls, and she had called for help. Ann Marie did not want to call us, but the roommate felt they should so she took the initiative. The person from the state reassured Ann Marie that she was doing everything right and apparently gave her encouragement. Cindy by that time was calm, and we did what we could to work through the situation with both the girls.

A few days later, the roommate moved out, citing as her reasons not only Cindy's behaviors but also having to share a bathroom with her. Boy did we see that one coming, but no one listened to us. It turned out to be very convenient for Ann Marie as her boyfriend started spending more and more time at the house and eventually was pretty much living there. We were not entirely thrilled about that as we did not know him, but once again, we were told by the folks at the state we did not have much say in it. And they continually told us, "Providers are hard to find." He seemed nice enough, but we had a problem because the house revolved around him and not Cindy. For instance, Cindy would eat dinner very late because Ann Marie wanted to wait for her boyfriend to get home. Despite this, things still progressed fairly nicely for the next few months.

Chapter 8
FACILITATED COMMUNICATION

About four or five months after Cindy moved into her home, I attended a conference on facilitated communication. This is a method that originated in Australia and was introduced in this country by a highly recognized and respected professor at Syracuse University. I knew of him and his reputation and attended several of his conferences and respected him. He is a world-renowned advocate for people with disabilities and for inclusion. He was very involved in the move to close local institutions and build more community-based programs and individualized services.

Facilitated communication (FC) involves a person called a facilitator assisting a person with a disability to spell out messages either on a board or on an electronic device by giving support. In the beginning, the facilitator may provide support by holding the person's hand in theirs to help with the initiation but not actually to move the hand. The facilitator is supposed to provide some light resistance. The intent is to eventually fade that support so the person is communicating entirely on their own. It was something new and exciting, and I hoped it would be something Cindy could use. There were incredible stories of discoveries of people who have autism and were thought to be profoundly retarded who were now able to type highly intelligent thoughts. Their personalities and true potential were discovered. No one was ever able to explain exactly why the method worked, but it was thought to help with the inability to initiate. Indeed, some of the success stories were legitimate as some folks were able eventually to type with the only support being the facilitator's hand on the person's shoulder. But others still required a hand-in-hand support and therefore left the method open to considerable skepticism.

At the conference, I spoke with the keynote speaker, who was the woman who originated this method. I briefly told her about Cindy and asked if she thought this method would be useful to her. Her response was that their success with people who are deaf was very limited but that I should give it a try anyway.

I had mentioned the conference and my conversation to Ann Marie. Because she was a student studying special education at Syracuse University, I have no doubt she knew about FC. It was the talk of the town and the subject of many newspaper articles and television shows. ABC Television's Diane Sawyer did a story about it on one of the evening shows. She interviewed many people in Syracuse, including families, professionals, and people with disabilities. Some of them were the children of parents I knew well. I felt that if they said this was real for their children, I should not doubt that. So I decided I would look into finding someone to work with Cindy on it and told Ann Marie of my intent to do that.

CINDY IS FACILITATING?

Without my knowledge, Ann Marie decided to try this on her own even though she did not have the required training recommended to be a facilitator. She called me one day in January and said Cindy had facilitated with her on her first attempt. I was surprised she got a response so quickly because my understanding was that it could take considerable time even for a person who could hear. When I asked her what she had been facilitating, she told me she knew her colors and had been facilitating those. That did not surprise me at all because Cindy had known her colors for some time and would easily sign them when asked. She also told me she facilitated about a teacher at St. Mary's whose name started with a "D." I said yes, she had a teacher for many years that Cindy adored, and her sign name was done with a "D." I did not give it much more thought and did not think there were any great revelations as yet. Everything she was telling me were things Cindy could easily sign. Ann Marie suggested I come over the next night to witness this myself. I told her I would love to see this but that night we had tickets to a show. Cindy was coming home the following night for dinner, and I suggested she could show me then.

Two nights later, Cindy was home for dinner and we had a lovely time with her. She appeared to be very happy to spend the time with us. After dinner, Ann Marie came to pick her up, and I asked about the FC. Ann Marie told me Cindy had been up most of the night facilitating and had to stay home from school because she was so exhausted. When I seemed surprised and asked what she had been facilitating, Ann Marie just smiled with a cocky sort of grin. I probably did not seem very enthusiastic because everything I had learned about FC led me to believe that it was most likely a lengthy process. I tried to be supportive but continued to ask what she had been facilitating, and Ann Marie continued to grin.

"Cindy likes country music," she finally said.

"How can that be when she can't hear it," I replied.

Ann Marie just stood with that same smug grin on her face and said nothing. I continued to ask how that could be, and she continued not to respond.

"Are you trying to tell me that Cindy is not deaf?" I asked.

"Cindy is not ready for you to know that yet," she replied after a brief hesitation and with a smile on her face.

"Perhaps you have become overzealous in your efforts. I think you should step back," I said calmly and politely after taking a deep breath.

"I know this is scary and upsetting for you," she said.

"We have already identified a graduate student who is trained and willing to try this with Cindy. I want you to stop it," I spoke in a calm but firm voice.

Ann Marie was obviously very angry with the suggestion and gathered up her belongings and Cindy and left without saying another word to me.

"I appreciate your efforts and am sorry if I upset you but I feel it best you not continue the facilitation," I said as she was walking out the door. I felt bad that she was angry but thought she would get over it.

The next morning, I spoke with Cindy's case worker at the state, Sarah. I told her what had happened, and we even joked about Cindy not being disabled and losing all her services. We also laughed about how ridiculous it was to think Cindy wasn't deaf. I also called Ann Marie and asked if we could get together and talk about what had happened. I felt bad that she was upset and wanted to work things out. She agreed to talk and said she would get back to me but never did.

That same day, Ann Marie called the state offices and said Cindy needed to see them immediately. Sarah and a psychologist, Kristen, went to Cindy's house where they observed Ann Marie and Cindy facilitating. That same afternoon, Bob picked up Cindy to come home for the weekend, and Kristen was still there. It appeared to Bob that Cindy was angry at Kristen, who was restraining Cindy's hands. Bob had no idea what had taken place. Cindy went willingly with her father and had a great weekend home with us. She was very happy to be home.

OUR NIGHTMARE BEGINS

The following Monday I received a call from the head of the children's team at the local state office saying they wanted to visit us and would be there the next day. I was somewhat nervous about this and spoke to a fellow parent and friend about it. She agreed it was highly unusual and thought something serious must have happened. That afternoon, Nanette, the woman who called me, and Bill, another administrative person, came to see me. They were both people I already knew and had sat on committees with and otherwise dealt with for years. After the initial pleasantries, I asked what was going on. Bill told me they had received a call from Ann Marie that Cindy was facilitating and was not deaf. I was somewhat shocked it had gotten that far.

"You don't really believe that do you?" I asked.

"We do believe it. Cindy was observed facilitating with Ann Marie. Cindy has stated she is not deaf and not retarded but has been faking it her entire life." I could not believe my ears but there was more.

"Cindy also facilitated her father sexually abused her."

"What? You cannot be serious? You are not really buying this nonsense, are you?" I asked with anger.

They told me they were perfectly serious and they did believe Cindy was facilitating and that she was indeed not deaf nor retarded and has been faking it. They also added they were not convinced she was being truthful about the sexual abuse charge.

I reminded them that Cindy spent eight years at a school for the deaf where audiological tests were done frequently. I also told them that at age five she had had a BSER test done, which confirmed her deafness. Although they were not aware of that, they said they believed the tests could be wrong. I kept telling them that this whole thing was ridiculous and that Ann Marie did not know what she was doing. Furthermore, even the idea that her father would do such a thing both angered and insulted me.

"You know me. If there was the slightest chance of something like that, which there is not, I would throw Bob out on the street in two seconds."

I could not get over what they were saying and continued to disbelieve they were giving any credence at all to this absurdity. I pointed out that Cindy had just been home and was very happy and questioned how that could be. Why would she go willingly and eagerly with her father after saying such horrible things? Their explanation was that she had hidden the truth for so long and she was continuing to do so with us. It was her way of controlling her world.

While we were having this discussion, Bob came home from work. I told Bill and Nanette that they were going to have to tell him this, that I refused to even say the words. Bob told me much later that when he walked into that room and saw my face, he thought that Cindy had died. They repeated the story, and Bob was also in shock. After citing many of the same concerns and reasons for disbelief that I had, he began to defend himself.

"If Cindy is communicating, why she would say anything like that? I promise you at no time have I ever done anything to her."

I reassured him in front of Bill and Nanette that he did not have to defend himself and I knew there was no justification for this ridiculous accusation. They said the next step would be to bring in an expert in FC to verify that Cindy was indeed facilitating. I reluctantly agreed as I felt we had to do something to officially end this farce.

After they left, Bob and I were still in shock and spent most of the evening and late into the night talking, trying to figure out what was really going on. Apparently, the day after Ann Marie left our house angry, she made a phone call to OMRDD telling of the facilitation and the accusation of abuse. Even though Bob and I did not really believe Cindy was actually doing this, we could not help focusing on why she would ever say that. We questioned ourselves as to whether there could be any truth to the claim she could hear, and if even any part of this was true, why she would say such a thing. We talked about what could have possibly happened in the past that would warrant such an accusation.

We talked about how when Cindy was young, Bob often helped lift her out of the bathtub. Could he have accidentally brushed her breast while doing that, and she perceived it as abusive? It had been many years since he had done that as when Cindy became an adolescent, he no longer took care of personal needs out of respect for her. If he helped with her personal needs at all, it was only the rare occasion when he had no other choice. We just could not understand any of this or how anyone could even give any credence to it. It was such a confusing time. We still felt she was deaf but we continued to question what she was saying as if she wasn't.

WHAT DO WE DO NOW?

We didn't know what to think or do and felt we had to talk to someone about all of it. I told my brother who was very skeptical of this new method of communication and of course very supportive of us. We also told some close friends who were almost as shocked as we were. My girlfriend who knew about the meeting called me to find out what happened, and when I told her, she was just plain angry. She pointed out that FC was very new and untested. Yes, there had been remarkable discoveries, but many people were just plain caught up in it and not thinking clearly. She was a sharp parent who had her own share of difficulties advocating for her son and cautioned me to be very careful with this.

In a follow-up phone call with Nanette, I told her I wanted some proof this was coming from Cindy. Nanette was going to observe Cindy and Ann Marie and agreed to try to get some validation by asking casual questions about family members and such. That Friday she made that visit and called me after to give me a report. She asked about cousins, aunts, and uncles and what Cindy had done when she was home the previous weekend. All the names and information that Cindy gave were incorrect. That did not change Nanette's opinion at all, and she suggested we bring in an expert.

The following Monday, Nanette called to tell us that according to Ann Marie, Cindy had recanted her accusation of abuse. While we were relieved about that part, it did not lessen what we were feeling. I also told Nanette that I found out that the incorrect relative's names Cindy had given were the names of Ann Marie's relatives. Remarkably, that still did not change her opinion.

Bob and I also decided to talk with someone else who knew us well. Ronald is a clinical psychologist and a parent of a child with a disability. I had seen Ronald professionally on and off over the years to help me deal with the difficult times in our life, but both Bob and I knew him on a personal level as well. I made an appointment, and we both went to see him. Ronald was very familiar with FC and had been using it with his son. Even so, he recognized the impact of what was happening to us at the time and wanted to help us sort through it. He also told us we were the fifth family to come to him with this same problem.

The first thing Ronald did was to ask me to leave the room. Bob told me later that when I did, Ronald told him that anything he said would remain confidential between the two of them. He needed Bob to be truthful with him and asked him if he ever did anything to Cindy. Bob told me that he gave him an emphatic no and recounted our conversation of possible reasons she would say these things. I was called back in, and we talked about what to do next. Ronald was a friend of a professor who was very familiar with FC and asked our permission to speak with him about this. He thought he could suggest someone to determine whether Cindy was actually facilitating.

OH MY GOD, THIS IS REALLY HAPPENING!

A few days later, it was decided that Timothy, a speech pathologist, would visit Cindy and Ann Marie to determine if the facilitation was indeed happening. Nanette and Bill from OMRDD would also be there. My biggest mistake was not being there also. Even though Cindy had supposedly recanted her accusations of abuse,

I was so angry at Ann Marie and so very uncomfortable about the whole thing that I didn't go. It was agreed I would be called at the conclusion of the meeting. It was a Friday afternoon, and Deb was spending a weekend away at a respite house. It was supposed to be a weekend of fun and relaxation for us, but I was a nervous wreck.

In the early evening, I got the call and was told by Nanette that Timothy had observed Cindy and Ann Marie and declared that Cindy was truly facilitating. In addition, Cindy had facilitated with Timothy that she was sorry she lied about the abuse. Nanette pointed out that because Timothy had no prior knowledge of that accusation that it was the validation we were looking for. I spoke to Timothy myself, and he confirmed that he also had facilitated briefly with Cindy. All of this was done by putting Cindy's hand with her index finger pointed in the palm of the facilitator's hand. Timothy told me Cindy said something about a noisy Halloween party and asked if I remembered that. I told him I didn't know of any Halloween party but that she might have been to one at St. Mary's. I was overcome with shock. Timothy also confirmed that while facilitating with him, Cindy stated she lied about the abuse against her father and was sorry for it. I was grateful that was no longer an issue.

I was alone when I got the call and cried like never before. When Bob came home and I told him, he could not believe it. I called Ann Marie and asked if we could come over and see Cindy. She protested saying she was tired but I insisted. After all, if what they were saying was true, I finally had a chance to have a conversation with my daughter, something I had always dreamed about. We went there on the premise that we believed it was happening, although I know it had not yet sunk in.

"Has anyone ever physically hurt you?" was my first question. Because Cindy had been away so much, it always nagged at me. She assured me no one had.

"Do you know how much we love you?" She said she did. It was intensely emotional as we "spoke" with Cindy through Ann Marie. There were so many things we wanted to ask her and tell her.

Some things she said just did not make sense, such as she did not like shrimp. She has always loved shrimp, and we would have to hold back the platter or she would eat the whole thing. Earlier with Nanette, Cindy told her she had chicken for dinner when she was home and a large bowel movement. Neither was correct, but we were told it was not unusual for people to lie.

HOW COULD WE HAVE BEEN SO WRONG ALL THESE YEARS?

That night at Cindy's, both Bob and I were in tears. We had been told that the facilitation was real and we were supposedly communicating for the very first time with our daughter. I cannot adequately describe our feelings. We were trying to absorb and believe what we were being told, but at the same time it was so overwhelming. It was wonderful because we could communicate and awful because we had wronged Cindy so. We wanted so desperately for it to be true and yet dealing with that was unbearable. It was a time of incredible highs and devastating lows. Our dreams were coming true, and our life was being shattered, all at the same time.

We were also furious with Ann Marie's lack of sensitivity. Here we were at this time of incredible breakthrough, and she was rude and acted put out. Her boyfriend came strolling through the kitchen with a pizza and went about fixing his dinner like it was an ordinary day. Ann Marie was more interested in him. Cindy was more interested in the pizza. Their actions just didn't seem to fit the incredible revelations being made. The so-called experts were telling us Cindy was not deaf or retarded, and we desperately wanted that to be true. We believed what they were telling us, but there was still a nagging sense that something was not right. So many things did not make sense.

That night I completely broke down. I was totally hysterical, and Bob had a difficult time consoling me. To this day I do not know why we believed what they were telling us, but at that point we did. All these professionals were saying the same thing, and I guess both Bob and I succumbed to the pressure. Even Ronald, whom we highly respected, now believed what the others were saying. I was overcome by both shock and guilt. Ronald called me that same evening and spent hours on the phone with me trying to calm me and counsel me. All I could think of was that I had wronged Cindy terribly and would never be able to make it up to her. There were so many things going through my mind, memories of past experiences and how I should have done things differently. I even thought about small things, like all the times I softly mumbled angry words behind Cindy's back thinking she couldn't hear me.

While we were thrilled of course that Cindy could hear and was not retarded, that joy was dampened by the realization she had a whole set of different problems. The prospect of our actually being able to communicate with her was overshadowed by the realization that we had been so wrong about her for twenty years. Where did we go wrong and how could we have missed all this? We thought she must hate us so much to spend her life trying to deceive us. The explanation given to us was because she was brilliant and had so much to deal with early in life that this deception was her way of controlling things. Ronald tried to make me understand it was not my fault and that it was Cindy's doing, not mine. After some time, I agreed to continue my counseling in his office and made an appointment.

The next day Ann Marie called me and told me that Cindy had stayed overnight at a supervised apartment where Cindy did respite and showed Barb, a staff person, how to facilitate. I asked Ann Marie if she would call me and tell me some of the things Cindy said but she never did. The next day I got a call from Barb, who said she was in total shock and was thrilled Cindy could communicate. She said Cindy was pointing to letters and she thought she was trying to spell the word trouble but not hitting the letters exactly. Leslie, another resident, was causing trouble and Barb thought perhaps that was what Cindy was trying to spell. The following Monday, Ann Marie wrote in the school communication book that Cindy spelled out Leslie is a troublemaker. When I called Barb to verify that, she told me that was not true. Cindy did not spell anything.

GETTING HELP

Once again, Bob and I both went to see Ronald, and he helped us get through this awful experience, recognizing that our world as we had known it had been destroyed. He recommended I see a psychiatrist who could prescribe medication for post-traumatic stress. I agreed to do that but never got to it. We also talked about working with Timothy to try to get Cindy to facilitate with us so we could establish direct communication. We agreed to set up an appointment that next week to do just that. In the meantime, we would try as hard as we could to get Cindy to facilitate with us.

The next week, Timothy came to our home to talk with Bob and me and gave us a copy of Cindy's typings. He talked about FC in general and gave us hints to help us facilitate with Cindy. Cindy was going to spend a long weekend at home and Timothy would return that Monday night to help the process.

WHY WON'T SHE TALK TO US?

When Cindy came home for her weekend visit, she was the Cindy we always knew. She signed to us like always, acted the same as she always did, and seemed very happy to be home. If she was angry at us, she certainly was not showing it. She also never gave any indication that she could hear and still did not startle to a loud noise. We were told she might be reluctant to reveal herself to us. This was another thing that was so very difficult for us. Bob and I devoted our lives to her well-being and fought all her life to get others to believe in her. We were told she would be a vegetable. We refused to accept that. We saw much more in her and worked to get doctors to see it also. When she was misdiagnosed and others refused to work with her, we fought for her until people admitted they were wrong. Throughout her school years we advocated to get others to recognize her potential. We spent her entire life highlighting her abilities and showing them to others. Why would she reveal herself to a virtual stranger and not us? How could she have ever thought we did not believe in her?

Over the weekend, we made every effort to try to facilitate with Cindy, with absolutely no progress. Every time we tried, she became agitated so we did not push it. We talked with her constantly and tried our best to reassure her that we loved her. We were still in shock that Cindy was able to pull off this deception. We couldn't understand how she could have faked everything, including the hearing tests and even her lack of a startle reflex. I was assured by the folks at the state that all of this was possible. Despite everything that was happening and my mental state, we had a very nice few days with Cindy. If indeed she hated us, she was still covering it well and we were having a hard time believing it was true. No matter what we did, Cindy continued to act like a person who is deaf.

Bob and I spent hours day after day re-examining our life since Cindy was born. We questioned every decision and so many of Cindy's actions. We still could not understand how all this could be real. So many things still did not make sense, but the professionals kept telling us it was possible. We thought about different things Cindy had done over the years. For instance, one evening while I was out, Bob had been working in the yard spreading mulch. Feeling kind of dirty, he decided to take a very quick shower. He locked all the doors and made sure both the girls were settled and occupied. He got into the shower and quickly out again and immediately checked on the girls. Deb was still occupied, but Cindy was not where she had been. He started searching the house only half-dressed when the doorbell rang. As soon as he opened the door, he realized it was unlocked. A boy who lived down the street and rode the bus with Deb said that he had seen her sister. While questioning the boy, Bob took off running asking where she was. About a block away on a very busy street at dusk, he saw a group of people standing on the side of the road. The sense of panic overwhelmed him as he drew closer. Cindy was sitting on the ground surrounded by a woman and some teenagers. When he caught his breath, the woman asked if he was her father. She told him Cindy was walking down the middle of the road while cars honked their horns and swerved around her. She stopped her car and managed to get Cindy off to the side. Bob couldn't thank her enough and then proceeded to get Cindy back home. We never had any idea where she thought she was going. But we could not help but wonder how someone who was supposed to be able to hear and be so intelligent would be so reckless. It did not make sense.

We remembered dozens of times and experiences that no longer made sense if all this was true. Once when Cindy was young, we took her to the New York State Fair. At the time, we were working hard on her signing vocabulary, including food items and animals. She knew the signs for milk and cow, and we would sign to her that milk came from the cow. She would always repeat what we signed to her and still does to this day. While at the fair, we walked through the livestock barns signing the names of the animals. We came upon a milking demonstration and signed to her again that milk comes from the cow. As usual, she echoed in sign. When the farmer saw us, he motioned us over so she could see the pail and what he was doing. She looked in the pail and signed milk with a huge grin. The look of surprise on her face was priceless. It was one of those rare and wonderful teachable moments. Now we were being told that was faked.

CINDY FACILITATES WITH US

When Timothy came, we all sat in the family room, with Cindy sitting in her favorite armchair. Timothy sat on her left on a chair taken from the kitchen. Timothy had brought a Canon communicator that produced a tape of what was typed. Timothy, holding Cindy's hand completely in his, began facilitating immediately with Cindy.

"How are you tonight?" Timothy asked.

"I am excited to be here and have a lot to talk about with my mom and dad."

With tears in my eyes, I said I was glad because I had questions about so many things and I was so grateful to actually be able to talk with her. Timothy instructed me to frame my questions carefully.

"Do you want to talk about the past, the present, or the future?" Timothy asked.

"I want to talk about the future and how it affects me," Cindy spelled.

While it was not exactly what I wanted, at least it was communication. This was something both Bob and I had longed for since Cindy was born. We had always said that we would sell our souls to be able to have a conversation with her, and as difficult as the situation was, our dream was becoming a reality. It was the opportunity we had hoped and prayed for, and we were about to embark on a journey we never thought would happen. That part of it at least was incredibly thrilling.

At one point, Cindy spelled out a statement that I had to ask her to repeat. It was so profound that I told her I was not even sure what it meant. I did not pursue it because Timothy had told me he would send us a copy of all the communicator's printouts.

Conversation flowed freely between Timothy and Cindy. Cindy facilitated that she wanted to live alone, drive a car, and go to college. She also facilitated she wanted Timothy to teach her parents how to facilitate with her.

Timothy eventually asked Cindy if she would like to facilitate with her parents. Cindy responded that she would and wanted to have her father try first. Bob sat in the same chair that Timothy did, with Timothy right by him. He positioned Cindy's hand in Bob's and then supported them both with his. Cindy began facilitating immediately, again talking about going to college. I did not know what to think at that point. It appeared to me that Cindy was facilitating with her dad, and she had a huge smile on her face.

All the time this communication was taking place, Deb was playing with her toys on the floor in the same room. At one point, Deb wound up a small musical toy that was very soft and quiet.

"How do you like Debbie's music?" Timothy asked.

"Very much," Cindy facilitated. If it was truly her spellings, her hearing was excellent.

Timothy resumed as facilitator, and conversation flowed freely between him and Cindy.

The movement of facilitation is consistent back-and-forth motions, almost like that of sitting in a rocking chair. At one point, I looked over at Cindy, and while she was moving her hand, her eyes were closed and she appeared to be dozing. I asked her if she was tired. Timothy looked at Cindy and immediately put his free arm on Cindy's leg, and Cindy jerked slightly and opened her eyes. I was immediately suspicious at this point but unsure of what to do about it. I continued observing without saying anything. Bob was not in the room at the time, as he needed to attend to Deb, so he did not witness what I did.

Timothy asked Cindy if she would like to try it with me, and Cindy said yes. I sat in the same chair, and once again he positioned Cindy's hand in mine and supported us both with his. We also started facilitating immediately, but as soon as we did, I knew what was happening. There was absolutely no doubt in my mind that Timothy was guiding my hand, and the movements were his and not Cindy's. At one point, there was nothing but jumbled letters, and Timothy asked if I saw the pattern. He said it was the word chair. I saw no resemblance.

Another time, Cindy was supposedly trying to spell living, and Timothy asked if I could see where she was going. I said I thought so, and Timothy instructed me to anticipate and help her. I started moving Cindy's hand myself toward the letters to spell the word room, and Timothy said, "That's it, Mom. You've got it." I was livid but did not want a confrontation right there. I was so nervous inside as I did not know what Bob had experienced and so I said nothing. My heart was pounding so hard I thought I was going to have a heart attack. My initial reaction was to jump up and throw him out. I was incredibly angry but held it in as I felt the need to be cautious. It was as if someone had declared war, and I had to maintain a sharp mind and carefully consider every move.

Timothy resumed as a facilitator for a while, and Cindy spelled out that she enjoyed being home for her visit and that she liked sleeping in her old bed and eating my food.

"Thank you. Which meal did you like the best?" I asked.

"I liked the barbecued chicken and mashed potatoes," Cindy replied.

I told Timothy we didn't have that. He then asked Cindy why she said that. Cindy replied that she didn't like being a guinea pig and so she lied. Timothy instructed me to frame my question by providing two or three of the things that we had to eat, all of which would be correct.

"Did you like the fish, pot roast, or the Spanish rice?" I asked.

"I liked the fine fish," Cindy replied. That was very interesting because we never had any of those things, but again, I kept that to myself. Timothy talked to Cindy about the confusion caused by lies and the need for her to just express her feelings.

I asked Timothy what he thought the next step should be, and he suggested we continue to facilitate with Cindy. He also offered his services to work with the folks at the school to help them become facilitators. Of course, this would be on a consultant basis, and he would charge the district. In fact, he had told us in our first meeting that becoming a consultant in this area was his goal. Timothy lectured us on the importance of not trying to trick or test Cindy. The questions should have choices, all of which should be correct answers. Very convenient.

Bob and I both saw Timothy to the door. After he left, I looked at Bob and said, "Well?"

"What do you think?" he asked.

We went back and forth a few moments with our hesitation, each of us not wanting to influence the other.

"I think he was moving my hand," he finally said as he looked at me with question.

"He was most definitely moving mine, and this whole thing is a crock of shit."

OUR TURNAROUND

We both spent a great deal of time that night talking about what had happened. Also, just to be absolutely sure, we tried to facilitate with Cindy again and of course got nothing. It was a major turning point for us. Somewhere in this whole mess, Bob and I forgot what we had learned over and over for so many years. We know Cindy better than anyone and we need to trust our instincts. Cindy is deaf, and she was not facilitating. I told Bob about the point where Cindy was falling asleep. We did not know why anyone was choosing to believe this or why Timothy was supposedly communicating but we were certain it was not happening.

We questioned how we could have been pulled into all of this and allowed people to tell us these bizarre things. Perhaps it just happened at a time in our life when we were incredibly tired. We had been through so much over the last twenty years, and it had not been that long since our bitter battle with the school district. Perhaps it was also our deep and passionate desire to be able to communicate with Cindy and our dream for her to be able to hear and be "normal." For that short period of time of probably a couple of weeks, we went through hell blaming ourselves because we believed what the so-called experts told us. But that was over, and we were convinced this facilitation was not happening.

Chapter 9
WE FIGHT FOR CINDY

I was no longer depressed; now I was just plain mad. We were raked over the coals and dragged through the mud because of a new, untested, and highly controversial method that no one really understood. Timothy's visit caused us to do a complete 180-degree turn.

I went immediately into my planning mode. We decided that for the time being we would let Timothy and everyone else continue to think that we believed Cindy was indeed facilitating so we would have time to gather information. Timothy was to send us a report that included the tape of the conversation as well as his recommendations. I wanted to make sure I got that report and the copies of the transcript and felt it important he thought I was on board until I received them. It was deceptive but I did not care. I felt like I was fighting for Cindy's life all over again. It was incredibly difficult. During that time, Ann Marie came to our house several times with Cindy. Cindy had supposedly facilitated that she wanted to come over for dinner. This FC became very convenient for Ann Marie, as Cindy would supposedly facilitate that Ann Marie needed respite, and Cindy would then spend the weekend with us or in a group home.

One night, Ann Marie came to pick up Cindy, who had spent the afternoon with us and had dinner with us also. We had a wonderful time, and Cindy was in excellent spirits. Shortly after she arrived, Ann Marie quickly scribbled the alphabet onto a piece of paper. Holding the flimsy paper in her left hand in midair and holding Cindy's hand in her right, Cindy starting facilitating. They were standing in the kitchen near the refrigerator, and Cindy had her head turned back trying to see what Bob was getting out of it. She could not see the paper, but this of course was not supposed to be unusual for FC. Cindy supposedly spelled out that her father did not believe in her, and she did not think he loved her. She also spelled that her father hurt her and she was very angry at him. All the time Cindy was supposedly saying these horrible things about her father, she was staring at Bob with a huge smile. Bob was getting food out of the refrigerator and showing it to Cindy. It was so obvious she was much more interested in him than what Ann Marie was doing. Cindy also seemed annoyed with Ann Marie, and she only responded to her when she used sign language. It was all I could do to keep from strangling Ann Marie.

During those weeks, Cindy supposedly facilitated many things, including that she wanted to study drama as well as Egyptian hieroglyphics. Cindy spelled out the latter when she and Ann Marie were visiting one time. Later, I went and looked up the spelling and found that Cindy, or I should say Ann Marie, had spelled it correctly. One day Cindy would say she wanted to attend Notre Dame and another day it was LeMoyne College. She also supposedly said she wanted to study anthropology as well as act and sing in musicals. Ann Marie told me that Cindy facilitated in the presence of her parents and that the things she said made them both laugh and cry. She often told us that Cindy was hurting because we did not believe in her. And even though the abuse charges had been recanted, they continued to be discussed and brought up again. Much of what she supposedly said could not be validated because it was not verifiable information. Those times she did facilitate verifiable information, it always proved to be incorrect.

When we finally got the report from Timothy, we found it interesting that the very profound statement I had asked him to repeat and said I didn't understand was not included in the transcript. I seriously considered calling Timothy to ask why but felt it would do no good.

PLEADING OUR CASE

Our first course of action was to contact Tom, the assistant director at the local state office, and set up a meeting. We had no childcare for Deb, so she went with Bob and me. I took with me all the records I had regarding Cindy's hearing tests, as well as educational records. I presented them to Tom and told him of our experience with Timothy. I also told him that we felt threatened by the accusations, even though they had been recanted, and saw all of this as a personal attack on us. We wondered if we should seek legal advice. Even though Cindy had recanted her accusation against Bob, it was a serious matter. If it came up again, we would have to deal with that.

We were angry that we as well as Cindy's doctors were being called into question. We also didn't like that Cindy was constantly being called a liar. Yet never had anyone questioned or doubted Ann Marie or Timothy, nor did they seek to verify anything that came through facilitation. Everything that was said and done was automatically taken as real and true. I suggested that people were so caught up in this new discovery that their professionalism and training went out the window. He was understanding and said he would take everything into consideration, but in the meantime, we should try to keep our minds open to the possibility that this was happening.

The next day I received a call from Nanette asking how I was doing facilitating with Cindy. I laughed and told her I was not in the mood to play games anymore and I was sure she knew about our meeting with Tom. She said yes, she did but was surprised by it as she had understood our meeting with Timothy went very well. I told her Bob and I both felt the whole thing was bogus, but Nanette disagreed and had an excuse for every argument. Nanette said the BSER that Cindy had done confirming her deafness was fifteen years old and therefore unreliable. According to Nanette, the people at St. Mary's were also wrong. In her opinion, Cindy was so highly intelligent that she fooled even them. I reminded her that except for the recanting of her allegations that was facilitated with Timothy and being used as validation, there was not one piece of information that Cindy gave that could be verified. I told her I needed just one thing that could only come from Cindy before I would even consider the possibility. That had not happened. She and a psychologist from her office, Kristen, were going to visit Cindy and would try to get something. But I was informed that what had been discovered about people who facilitated was that if they feel they are being tested then they either refuse to answer or lie. Again, very convenient.

While talking with Nanette, I asked her to tell me the specific allegation Cindy had made against her dad. I could not believe what she said. Bob and I were racking our brains to pinpoint a time when Cindy could have misunderstood an action, but what she supposedly said was so much worse. It was incredibly graphic, horrendous, and disgusting. I do not know why it took me so long to ask, but it was probably because I knew it did not happen. I was also told Cindy called her father a "lame bastard" and blamed him for sending her away to Buffalo. After hearing all this, my anger intensified. I did not believe she said any of those things. Cindy adores her father, and he did not like the idea of her going to school in Buffalo. He agreed because we had no other choice. When I hung up the phone, I was livid.

MEETING WITH DOCTORS

At the same time, I quietly made some appointments. Although he was no longer her primary physician, I first visited one of her pediatricians as he had taken care of her for eighteen years. I told him about everything that had happened, including the abuse charge that had been recanted. He listened intently with a slight look of disbelief on his face. I told him that if this claim were true that not only would we as parents have been horribly wrong about Cindy, but he would have been also. Everything he had thought and done for Cindy would have been off base. When I finished, he said that this story was very interesting, especially since he had just recently attended a grand rounds session on FC. He told me what I was telling him was a completely different side to what he had heard there. I asked if it was physically possible for someone to fake a BSER test while they were sedated, or if an infant really could fake deafness and the lack of a startle response. He said that was highly doubtful. I believed he was somewhat angered by what I had told him, and he immediately called the neurologist that had seen Cindy a few years before. She also was surprised by what she heard and offered to work with us to get another BSER test done. I met with her later, and we decided that we would try to do the test as an outpatient, and she would prescribe a sedative for Cindy. She felt if Cindy were intelligent enough to study anthropology, then she could certainly sit still for a test. If for some reason they were unable to complete the test, then we might have to consider general anesthesia. Bob and I did not share with anyone that we were going to have this test done but chose instead to keep it to ourselves.

I also met with Cindy's current primary physician, an internist. I wanted her to know what was going on and how we were proceeding. I also wanted her to know our feelings about Ann Marie and that we were at odds with the people at the state. I asked her not to share anything with them without my permission. She agreed and she too was somewhat taken aback by what I had told her. I assured her I would keep her informed and make sure she received copies of all reports. I also contacted St. Mary's School for the Deaf to get copies of all her hearing tests, as well the clinic in Rochester that did the BSER.

While all of this was taking place, Kristen started seeing Cindy on a regular basis to "counsel" her, which I objected to and asked her to stop. Bob and I both are Cindy's legal guardians and therefore should have had some control over that. Kristen would not reveal anything Cindy supposedly said, citing confidentiality reasons. Kristen continued to counsel her even after she was instructed to stop. I ended up calling Tom and demanded he make her stop as she was using a method that had not yet been verified. I questioned who she was counseling, Cindy or Ann Marie? I pointed out the counseling was using a method that was in dispute. Fortunately, he agreed with me and ordered Kristen to stop the counseling sessions. I found out later she disobeyed those orders.

THEY DID NOT HAVE VALIDATION

We met again with Ronald and brought him up to date on what had been happening as he had been out of town for a few weeks. I believe he was somewhat surprised but never questioned what we told him. We told him we no longer believed the facilitation was real. We explained our many reasons why, including our experience with Timothy and the considerable incorrect information supposedly coming from Cindy. I told him the only thing I could not understand or explain was the validation the first night with Timothy where Cindy initiated conversation about the allegations. The people from the state were adamant Timothy had no knowledge of that and therefore could not have initiated it. That still puzzled me, and I had no explanation. It was then that Ronald told me that he had spoken with Timothy before he went to that session and told him of the allegations and the recanting of them. It was one of many times throughout the ordeal that the so-called professionals would fail to get facts before they jumped to conclusions. When I told people at the state that Timothy did have knowledge about the allegations, it still did not change their opinion. But it certainly solidified it for us. Now there was not one piece of validation.

Ronald suggested we set up a meeting with Timothy to determine what happened. We did that and specifically told the DSO we did not want Kristen there, and she was instructed by her superior to stay away. She showed up anyway, and the meeting was not pleasant. We confronted Timothy and told him we felt he was moving our hand. He became upset and indicated he was insulted by the accusation. We had a very intense meeting, but in the end, all agreed that the big question was whether Cindy was deaf. Everyone agreed that for the facilitation to have been real, she would have to have been able to hear. The way she was positioned with Timothy at our house, as with others, she could not possibly be lip-reading. Ronald asked Timothy how he would feel if it was determined that Cindy was indeed deaf and therefore could not be facilitating. He said he would have to re-examine his life as it was now.

It was agreed that people would continue to look at this and find a way to test Cindy. The idea of repeating the BSER had already been suggested by Nanette at the DSO. While I was not opposed to the idea, my concern was putting Cindy through something that might traumatize her. It was possible she might have to be put under general anesthesia to do the test and that was a risk.

I suggested that there could be other testing done, simple things like trying to get verifiable information. That suggestion, of course, was met with the standard excuse that people who facilitate do not like being tested and very often do not cooperate. One solution suggested by Kristen was for Cindy to practice the test. I objected to this, and after some discussion, it was agreed not to "practice" and not to alert Ann Marie to the questions. The meeting was an extremely tense one. When Timothy put on his insulted act, I told him Bob and I felt like we were fighting for Cindy's life and that we felt she was in an unsafe situation. Kristen kept defending Ann Marie and irritating me because she was not even supposed to be at this meeting. Also, Kristen was now claiming that Cindy was facilitating with her also on just a minimal basis. Directly after the meeting, without my knowledge or consent and against what had been agreed to, Kristen went directly to Cindy's and told Ann Marie everything, including the planned test. The three of them spent considerable time practicing.

A graduate student trained in FC was assigned to work with Cindy. She spent several sessions with Cindy trying to get her to facilitate but was unable to do so, although she said that despite her lack of success, she was convinced the facilitation was real. Her reasoning was that she could stand behind Cindy and ask a question and she would facilitate her answer with Ann Marie. The basis for FC was to assume it was real so no one would consider the fact that Ann Marie could hear the question. And there were never any questions to which Ann Marie would not know the answer.

It was so frustrating for us, and the lack of professionalism angered us tremendously. We asked for information from Cindy that could be verified. Over the course of a few months, there was not one piece of correct verifiable information. She could not correctly name relatives or tell what she had to eat while home or who came to visit her while she was at home with us. Every time I pointed out that what she was saying was incorrect, the explanation would be that she was lying.

THEY DID WHAT?

Shortly after Timothy's visit, I contacted Veronica at school to let her know what was going on. Not long after, Veronica called me to ask if I had given Ann Marie permission to sign papers on my behalf.

I said no and asked why. She told me that Ann Marie was signing official papers intended for me. In addition, she had requested that Cindy be signed up for some advanced courses being held at Syracuse University.

I was also told that Kristen had come to school and met with the principal to tell her that Cindy was not deaf, was brilliant, and should be removed from the special education program and put immediately into regular classes full time. I was so angry I thought I would burst. After Veronica calmed me down, she said she would arrange an immediate meeting with the principal.

I got off the phone with Veronica and immediately called Tom at the DSO and informed him of what was happening. Kristen was still disobeying direct orders, as well as going to the district when she had no right. I reminded him that Bob and I are Cindy's legal guardians. He assured me he would speak to those involved and that the counseling would stop.

The fact that Kristen would go to school in that way was a potential disaster. We still at that time had not settled the court case over Cindy's program. The district would have loved nothing better than to find out that Cindy was indeed not deaf. It would have taken them right off the hook, and they could have come back and sued us for damages. I cannot remember when I have been as angry as I was then. If they had listened to Kristen, we would have been right back to square one with the district. I must admit, however, that putting Cindy into regular classes was probably the last thing they would want to do.

I met at school with Veronica, the principal, and, of course, Kristen. It was an unpleasant meeting, and Kristen accused me of not being able to accept that Cindy was brilliant. I reminded everyone that as yet, there was not one piece of correct verifiable information to support the authenticity of this method. Fortunately, Veronica knew Cindy and me well enough and was smart enough to hold any decision until she herself could make an informed judgment.

At the end, the principal said it was obvious that Kristen and I were at odds about this matter, and her bottom line was that she had to answer to the parent and legal guardian. But she thought it would be worth further investigating the possibility. Veronica agreed to try FC with Cindy in the class. I also informed them that I would be bringing in an outside psychologist as well. It was coincidentally the year for Cindy's triennial evaluation required by law, and I did not want the school psychologists doing it.

TIME FOR TESTING

I contacted Michael, a psychologist whom I had previously worked with, to do testing for Cindy. He also worked at the DSO. I told him about everything that was going on and asked him during his testing to see if there was any indication Cindy was not deaf. He was not shocked by what was happening but reminded me of how serious a situation it was. Even though the abuse charges had been recanted, he told me that charges like that could destroy our lives. Bob could lose his job, and we could lose custody of Deb. What he said both frightened me and angered me even more. I told him I wanted him to look at this with as open a mind as possible to see if there was even an inkling of truth to any of it. He spent considerable time with Cindy both at our home and at school and observed her with Ann Marie as well. His bottom line was that he saw no indications that Cindy could hear, and her testing was consistent with what it had been in recent years.

Cindy attended a regular art class, although at one time with Ann Marie she supposedly facilitated she hated art. That was one of the many inconsistencies. Cindy has always loved doing arts and crafts activities. As in most regular classes, students had homework. Some was sent home with Cindy. When not returned, Ann Marie claimed she didn't see it until late. When told to do it whenever she could, Ann Marie replied Cindy didn't want to. Another homework assignment was sent, and the teachers were told that Cindy wanted the textbook to refer to. That was sent home with her. If the questions were based on the book and she had it, the answers were OK. But if the questions were based on the lecture in class, they were incorrect.

Veronica was also doing testing for the triennial and did so looking for indications Cindy was not deaf. Everything she did indicated there was no truth to any of this, and Cindy was not showing any signs of being brilliant.

To try to convince Kristen that the FC was not real, I suggested we perform some simple tests. Kristen and Cindy came to our house, and this time I had a video camera. We sat at the table and had several colored blocks in front of Cindy. Using sign language, I asked to her to pick up the red one, and she immediately did so and smiled at me. We did this several times with several items, always using sign language. Cindy was very cooperative. She seemed to be enjoying the test and continued to smile. We then repeated the same things without the use of sign or the ability for her to see our lips. There was no response. Kristen and I both tried to get Cindy to respond to anything without the use of sign, but no matter what we did, she would only respond to sign. When I asked Kristen why she thought that was, she claimed Cindy did not want to cooperate. This was so hard for me because no matter what we did, Kristen was not going to give up her claims that the FC was real and Cindy was not deaf.

Once when speaking to Michael, the psychologist, he told me about a conversation he had with Tom, the administrator at the DSO. He told Tom that he saw no evidence that Cindy could hear and that he did not think any of this was real. Tom told him that people in their office were staking their reputation on it being real, and Michael said he knew that and that it was too bad. Michael was one of the few professionals who looked at this in a clinical way and remembered his training.

WHY IS IT ALWAYS OUR PROBLEM?

One of the most difficult and frustrating things about what was happening was that during these months of dispute over FC, Cindy still lived with Ann Marie. Some people at the DSO thought Ann Marie was another Anne Sullivan who had made a miraculous discovery, while others were holding their opinions for the time being. To many people, I was the poor parent who they pitied because I had a problem. I was the one who could not accept that I had been wrong all these years and wanted Cindy to be retarded. People were constantly telling me how sorry they felt for me because I did not believe in my daughter. It was infuriating and had an all-too-familiar ring. It reminded me of years ago when I kept telling the professionals that Cindy was brighter than they were saying, and they told me I had a problem accepting the truth that she was hopelessly retarded. Now, I was trying to convince them she wasn't a genius as they were saying, and once again, I had a problem. First, I could not accept that she was retarded; now I could not accept that she was brilliant. How ridiculous that was. There was nothing we would have wanted more than for all of this to be true, but at the same time we only wanted it if it was truly authentic. Bob and I have often said we would sell our souls to be able to talk with Cindy. But that does not mean we would sell her soul.

CINDY IS COMMUNICATING WITH ACTIONS NOT WORDS

We were very worried at this point about Cindy. Her behaviors at her home had deteriorated considerably, which also cemented our feelings about everything that was happening. Eventually, the folks at school also started seeing some deterioration. Cindy started to wet her pants and not sleep well at night. All during this time, Ann Marie told everyone that Cindy had facilitated how grateful she was that Ann Marie came into her life, that if not for her she would have continued to keep her secret. Ann Marie pledged her undying friendship forever and at any cost, no matter what the circumstances. She vowed to stay in Cindy's life no matter what I thought of her. She gave Cindy a picture of herself and her boyfriend as a symbol of that bond. It sat on the top of Cindy's dresser. Bob and I were positively nauseated by all of this, but those who believed in FC thought she was a hero. We were the bad guys who were holding back and hurting our daughter.

Things began to not go so smoothly at Cindy's house, and Cindy began to lash out at Ann Marie as well as throw things and become destructive. Ann Marie used the FC to get additional respite, and Cindy started spending weekends at another home.

After one such weekend, Cindy's case worker at the DSO, Sarah, called me and told me that Cindy had facilitated with Mary, a staff person at one of the homes. Sarah told me she had talked directly with Mary and verified that Cindy did facilitate. I told her I found that hard to believe as Cindy had never met Mary before and questioned why she would do that with a stranger but not her parents. Sarah suggested I call Mary myself and speak with her. I did that and our conversation began with Cindy's general mood over the weekend, which had apparently been good. I told Mary I had been informed that Cindy facilitated with her and asked her what it was she had said. She said Cindy facilitated what she wanted for dinner. I asked if that was all and she said yes. I then asked Mary to describe the process and experience for me. She told me that she put three items on the kitchen table, a box of macaroni, a package of hot dogs, and a can of soup. Cindy pointed to the package of hot dogs. When I asked if she was supporting her hand at all, she indicated she was not and said Cindy pointed entirely on her own. After Cindy did that, Mary took her hand and together with Mary guiding they spelled out her choice by pointing to the letters on the board. Mary called this facilitated communication. It was a wonderful example of how people who really knew nothing about the process had gotten caught up in all the hype. Mary had no idea what FC was and her claim of Cindy facilitating was nothing more than someone trying to teach Cindy to spell. Cindy was very capable of pointing on her own and would frequently make choices. I do not believe Mary had any idea of the potential harm being done.

I called Sarah back and told her of my conversation, and she told me she had never thought about asking Mary to describe the situation. I had known Sarah for years and now she was in an extremely difficult place. Her superiors were still claiming the facilitation was real, and she was being torn so she stayed out of it as much as possible. But she did tell me one very interesting thing about the day Ann Marie first called the DSO and Sarah and Kristen went to Cindy's. When Ann Marie was facilitating with Cindy that day, she had Cindy's hand on top of hers, and it was Ann Marie's finger doing the pointing. Sarah questioned the position because it was not usually done that way, and after that, Ann Marie reversed the hand position. If she had not done that and others had observed the original positioning of the hands, perhaps it would never have gotten so far. That was not the way FC was usually done.

While Cindy's behaviors at her home were awful and getting worse every day, when she was at our house, she was just fine. When I pointed this out to the others and suggested Cindy was trying to tell us something, they refused to believe there was any meaning to it. They simply explained it as the stress of "coming out." It continually amazed and frustrated me that these so-called professionals were so caught up in this method that they threw their training and common sense right out the window. There continued to be many indicators the facilitation was not real and still not one thing to verify it was true. The decisive factor for us was that Ann Marie called us and told us that Cindy was having trouble with her bowel movements. We had noticed when she was home that she had very large movements. I spoke to Veronica and asked her to be on the alert and let me know what Cindy was doing at school.

It was only a short time later that we realized that Cindy had been withholding her bowel movements at home with Ann Marie but would have them at our house or at school. And we found out much later that Cindy even started withholding her urine also while in her home. This was a repeat of St. Mary's and told us Cindy was in real distress. She felt comfortable in our house or at school but not in her home with Ann Marie. As far as we were concerned, that was a strong and reliable message from Cindy.

THE TEST RESULTS

The appointment for the BSER test was in late March. We arranged for Cindy to come home for a visit. Although she was initially very nervous, Cindy did extremely well during the test and was very cooperative the entire time. It took a little while for the sedative to work, but eventually it did and the technician was able to complete the test. I was present the entire time and told I would receive the results in a week or so. Cindy's time at home with us was very pleasant, and she was very happy to be with us. The first week in April, Bob and I took a trip to Ocean City, New Jersey, to celebrate a birthday. Beforehand, while Cindy was home, we showed her brochures and told her our plans. We have always used both sign language and voice when we speak to her and we continued to do so. We were purposely giving her information to see if any of it came back through facilitation, although we were confident it would not. The day after we returned from our trip, the results of the test came in the mail. As we expected, the test showed that Cindy had a severe to profound hearing loss in both ears. While we were thrilled that we finally had proof that could not be disputed, it was again difficult to read the report. There was always that nagging hope in our hearts that Cindy wasn't deaf and would be able to speak to us someday. But we knew that would not be, and now we could put an end to this nonsense. Even though we expected the result we got and hoped it would put an end to the current trauma, it was in many ways difficult. It brought back all the feelings we had the first time we found out she was deaf. But reading that report also unleashed incredible anger in both Bob and me. We were furious that we and especially Cindy had been put through this nightmare. Coincidentally, the day the report arrived, we were to pick Cindy up at her house to come home overnight as it was her twentieth birthday and we had a special celebration planned for her.

IT GETS UGLY

When I arrived at Cindy's house, Ann Marie and Kristen were there, once again, counseling Cindy. I was instantly irritated and reminded Kristen she had been instructed by her superior to stop. She said she could not abide by that as Cindy needed her and she would continue on her own time if necessary. I sarcastically asked what Cindy had been facilitating this time and I was told it was confidential. I asked if Cindy told her that we had gone on a vacation, and Kristen said Cindy had indeed told them that. When I asked if she told them where, they indicated she had facilitated we had gone to someplace in western New York State. When I told them that was not correct, Kristen looked at Cindy, shook her head, and told her she had to stop lying all the time. I laughed and said I thought Ann Marie was the liar, not Cindy. Kristen shook her head again and told me how sorry she felt for me and that she felt Cindy really wanted to facilitate with me. She asked me to please try it again. I was feeling a little smug and nasty at the time so I played along.

I sat next to Cindy, smiled at her, and took her hand. Of course, I got nothing. Then Kristen sat next to me and put her hand under mine and began moving it. I immediately stopped and told her she was moving my hand, to which she replied that she was merely giving guidance as she knew what Cindy was going to say. I told her that was enough and asked her sarcastically if Cindy had told her what she had done with me a couple of weeks before when she was home. When she said no, I told both Kristen and Ann Marie that we had gone for another BSER. Kristen shook her head again and looked at Cindy.

"Oh Cindy, you shouldn't keep these things to yourself," Kristen said.

I then told them both that the reason Cindy didn't tell them is that she can't because the FC wasn't happening. The test confirmed that she is deaf and this whole thing is a sham. Kristen said that she did not believe that and that Cindy was faking the test just as she had done before.

I described our appointment and told them how cooperative she was and how she was sedated during the test, as well as how happy she was to spend time with us. Kristen then looked at me and spoke.

"I pity you. You are missing so much because you refuse to believe in Cindy. You can't accept that she can hear and that she is brilliant. I feel sorry for Cindy because you have hurt her so deeply." Her comments angered me so much that I started screaming at Kristen and Ann Marie.

"If this doesn't stop immediately, you are going to be in big trouble," I screamed, along with several other angry comments. It was an ugly scene. I admit I lost control.

Kristen suggested that perhaps it would be best if I took Cindy and left. Because Cindy could obviously see how upset I was, for once I felt Kristen was right. I gathered up Cindy's things and was ready to go. Before I did Ann Marie, walked up to me and looked me in the eye.

"You scare the hell out of me," she said.

"Good," I replied.

ANN MARIE MOVES OUT

When Cindy and I got home, I told Bob what had happened. Because it was Cindy's birthday, we decided to put it aside and focus on our celebration. It was late on a Friday afternoon by then, so there was no time to contact anyone at the DSO anyway. That would have to wait until Monday. Bob and I both, however, wondered how Ann Marie was going to react.

The next day Bob drove by Cindy's house to see if there was any activity. What he saw was Ann Marie in the process of moving out. Cindy was supposed to return to her home later that day, and Bob went over again to confirm that she was indeed gone. Then I called the emergency number at the DSO to tell them there was no one at Cindy's house and that her family care provider had unexpectedly moved out. They told me there was nothing they could do about it then.

I called the DSO the next day to find out what arrangements they were going to make for Cindy. Tom informed me that because Cindy was safe under our care, they did not have to provide an emergency placement for her. I objected to this and was told they would look for a placement but they doubted it would be soon.

It took almost nine months before she moved back into her house. During that time, Cindy remained at home with us with no services and little to no respite for us while we continued to pay all the expenses on an empty house. We were not pleased. We also found out later they knew AnnMarie was going to move out but never told us. As soon as we took Cindy home that weekend, they were off the hook.

We sent copies of the BSER to the DSO, and incredibly, Kristen still challenged it. She even went as far as to call the neurologist who read the test and wrote the report. He was a supporter of FC but assured her the report was accurate and Cindy could not hear.

I spoke with Nanette, and when I asked her what she thought after reading the test report, she responded saying she believed the report but still thought Cindy was facilitating. I could not believe my ears. Very shortly after that, I was informed that Cindy's case was being changed to another team, and we would no longer be dealing with either Kristen or Nanette. To me, it was obvious they were being taken off the case because they had really messed up, but no one ever came out and admitted that. Also, at no time did anyone from the DSO ever apologize to us for any part they played in what we had been through. The closest we ever got to an apology was a statement many years later in an entirely different situation from Tom. He admitted that we had been dragged through the mud and raked over the coals. And that did not even address what Cindy had been put through.

We never heard from Ann Marie again. She gave the keys to the house to someone at the DSO. Despite her vow to be Cindy's friend no matter what, Ann Marie left without ever saying goodbye to Cindy. The picture she gave Cindy was also gone, and we will never know if she took it with her or if Cindy destroyed it in anger. Cindy has never had any further contact with Ann Marie, which is just fine with us, and I don't think Cindy misses her at all. Nonetheless, when Ann Marie left, some people at the DSO still thought she was an unsung hero and we were still parents with a problem.

Shortly after we received the test results, we met again with Ronald. He set up a meeting with the professor who referred Timothy to discuss what had happened to us. He never challenged the BSER report and said that the FC could not have been happening because Cindy was deaf. He agreed it was a nightmare. When I asked how he explained Timothy's so-called facilitation, he admitted he did not have an answer for that but suggested I contact him to discuss it. I told him I would think about it, but at that point in time, I just wanted never to hear about FC again and could not have cared less about Timothy.

CAN THIS BE HAPPENING TO SOMEONE ELSE ALSO?

Shortly after that meeting, I read an article in the newspaper about a lawsuit involving FC. A girl using FC had accused her father of sexually abusing her and there was going to be a trial. Of course, there were no names of the family in the article, but it did give the names of the attorneys. The article focused on how FC was not an approved means of communication in the courtroom. Proponents of FC were trying very hard to get it to be accepted, and by this time, FC had been much publicized and was highly controversial. I had no way of knowing whether there was any merit at all to the case but I couldn't get my mind off of it. It was so familiar, and right in the same community. It was like someone had written our story and just changed the names, it sounded so similar. But this story went even further because the father had been removed from the home. The truth was, if things had gone a little differently, it could very well have been us in those headlines.

I agonized for a couple of days and finally decided to call the attorney. I was able to get through to her despite not giving my name and told her how the article touched me and why. She was very skeptical at first, questioning whether I was genuine because I wouldn't give her my name. I explained that I was a parent and it was a small community. I had to live here and unfortunately still maintain a relationship with these people. She asked me some questions about my experience, and I told her about what had happened, including the supposed verification by Timothy. When she heard that she asked me to please meet and talk with her as Timothy was going to be called as an expert witness in her trial. I agreed and went to see her. She was working with another attorney on the case. I wasn't especially crazy about her or her style, but the other attorney was very nice. She had been called in on this case because she made her living defending pedophiles. She said she had her reasons for doing that and didn't feel the need to defend herself, but in this particular case, she was certain the dad was innocent. I brought some of the papers and reports from Timothy and retold my story. They asked if they could have a copy of his report and after some hesitation and editing of identifiable information, I agreed. They thanked me and wished me luck.

I never knew for sure what the outcome of that trial was or what happened to the parent. I will never know for sure whether I did the right thing. It is entirely possible I helped a child abuser, and that thought makes me shudder. But I'd rather think I helped end a gross injustice to another innocent family fallen victim to abusive FC. I can only hope that what I did saved another parent from some agony. I did see an article in the paper much later about a lawsuit that was filed against a teacher and a school district in our community. Parents were suing for damages from false accusations made through facilitated communication.

PLEASE NO, NOT AGAIN!

We thought the nightmare was over, but found out a year or so later it was not. After graduating from high school, Cindy was enrolled in a day program through a local agency. She had a volunteer job working in a classroom at the Jowonio School, an integrated preschool program. The Jowonio School was the site of many of the earlier success stories of FC, and many of the professionals involved with FC had associations with the school. I got a call one day saying that Cindy was facilitating with a staff member in her day program, and it was thought she was not deaf. I started shaking so hard I could barely stand. I was not about to let this happen again. I requested an immediate meeting of the parties involved. Apparently, Cindy's day program staff who made this claim had been talking with someone who saw her with Cindy at the job site. This person told Cindy's day habilitation staff that they had worked with Cindy previously and did not think she was deaf. This conversation took place either at or just after an FC conference. Cindy's alleged facilitation began immediately after. Once again, the staff person was claiming Cindy could hear normally.

We had a very intense meeting where a number of informal tests were done that showed no indication that Cindy could hear. The staff person still was not willing to concede that the FC was not happening. She would not reveal the name of the person who made the claim. After the meeting, I went home and wrote an extremely strong letter to the executive director of the agency. I stated that if they were to continue to serve Cindy, it would be on the condition they treat her as a deaf person and they stop all efforts to facilitate. Her primary means of communication was sign language, and I demanded they use it. I received a letter back from the director saying they would comply. I also received a letter from the staff person saying she would comply also, although she was not ready to admit she was wrong.

NOW DEB IS FACILITATING?

Shortly after Ann Marie moved out, we were told Deb was facilitating in school. This was being done without my knowledge or approval. She was pointing to animals, colors, and other objects correctly when asked while someone was holding her hand. I immediately put a stop to it; everything that had happened was still too painful. Deb is very capable of pointing on her own, and we were already investigating electronic communication devices for her. Stopping the facilitating may not have been the right thing to do, but there was no way I would put us in that position again.

WE FELT POWERLESS

Bob and I have been through a great deal with both our children, but the FC ordeal was in many ways the most difficult. We had dealt with life and death situations, major legal battles, and countless other problems, but this one nearly caused me to have a nervous breakdown. The roller-coaster of emotions was enough to make anyone ill. Our hopes and dreams were raised only to be shattered once again. All the feelings and emotions that we had dealt with so many years ago we experienced all over again. For a while, I forgot everything that I had learned from Cindy over the years, but once again she showed me the way. It was her actions and nonverbal communication that convinced us. The answers have always laid with Cindy, and this time was no different. We just temporarily forgot. No, we did not convince everyone, and there are some who would probably still make their claims. But many people who were involved or have learned of the experience since were taught a valuable lesson. Cindy was used by Ann Marie for a reason we will never know. Other people were so caught up in the process, they forgot to really look at Cindy.

What was so difficult throughout this ordeal was our powerlessness against the bureaucracy of the state. They called the shots. No matter how many times we demanded some kind of proof or validation, they had an excuse for not getting it. We had no control over what they did. They were not able to control what their employees did. Bob and I are not stupid people. Over the years, we have become knowledgeable about how to work within the system. We have learned to work effectively with a variety of professionals. But in spite of all that, we were helpless. Only because we had legal guardianship of Cindy were we able to stop them from removing her from special education classes and putting her into excelled university courses. And only because we eventually provided medical evidence that she is deaf did we stop the ongoing facilitation.

Despite our nightmare, I still believe that FC works for some individuals. When support is faded back to just a hand resting on a shoulder, there is no question in my mind that the typing is real because it is merely someone typing. But when the support involves holding the hand completely in the facilitator's, I remain skeptical and would have to have it proven to me. I do not doubt that it is happening for some. I have friends who are parents and whom I highly respect. If they tell me their child is facilitating, then I believe them. But in my opinion, the method just cannot be trusted unless there is real verification.

Much to my surprise, I received in the mail a request to submit testimony to a national committee that was set up to review FC. I believe they had received my name from the professor that was involved as he knew that despite my experience, I still believed FC worked for some individuals. I submitted that testimony relating the experience, my feelings as well as some recommendations. I knew one of the committee members. She has a PhD in special education and has a son with autism who uses facilitation. We both were presenting at a workshop once when she called me aside and told me she was the one who reviewed my testimony and she was very moved by it. Much later, I saw her again and asked what had happened with the committee. She told me the review committee was established by a group of people who favored FC, and the membership was heavily stacked with proponents. The study was completed but the report was never released.

Chapter 10
THE STATE INSISTS ON KEEPING CONTROL

While Cindy was at home with us, and we were waiting for the state to find another family care provider, we approached them once again with the idea of the private NFP agency taking over Cindy's house. The agency had a new executive director and was developing individualized supports based on person-centered planning. The services they were providing were very individualized, and they wanted to do some creative things. I was very involved with the agency and believed strongly in its philosophy. But once again, we were told they could not oversee Cindy's home as they were not an approved family care provider. Despite the willingness of the executive director to do what was necessary to become approved, the folks at the DSO for whatever reason said no. They insisted only the state could oversee Cindy's home.

At this time, we were able to get an occasional weekend of respite. Sometimes the girls went to the same place, and others times different places. When a bed was available at the home nearby where Cindy had stayed before, she would go there. Because of the level of care Deb needed, she always went to an intermediate care facility (ICF). These were highly staffed, state-certified homes for people with medical issues. There were a couple of ICFs in the area where Deb went and another where both the girls spent a weekend together. One was a very large and beautiful house that was home to eight people with very intensive needs, many of them in wheelchairs. In addition, they had a couple of respite beds. Cindy was clearly not happy there and did not like the environment. Deb, who is so easygoing, basically just vegetated. I believe she was pretty much left to herself because she was so complacent. It wasn't that it was a bad place or that the staff was unkind, but it was a mini-institution and there were just too many people there to care for. My observations firmed my belief that congregate care —that is, a group home, — was not what I wanted for my daughters, and it definitely was not what they wanted either.

CINDY MOVES BACK TO HER HOME

After eight months of Cindy living at home, we were contacted by our case worker at the DSO. She told us they had a potential family care provider, and a meeting was set up for us to meet her. Patty worked for the state and knew Cindy from some of her respite, and we had some experience with her also. We considered this a benefit as she was very aware of some of Cindy's challenging behaviors. Patty had a good deal of experience in the field and an easygoing calm nature, and she was not easily flustered. We talked for a time about why we set up the house and how we wanted it to be Cindy's. We wanted Cindy to be able to have the freedom she wanted without all the rules of a group home. For example, Cindy always slept with the door open, but in the group home, it had to be closed. We also wanted her to have more choices in her life. Also, the things in the home would be hers, and if she destroyed them, she would be destroying her things, not someone else's. We had gotten many requests over the years from people looking for reimbursement because Cindy had destroyed something of theirs. We also told Patty that Cindy has always loved dogs and we would like her to have one, but she would need help taking care of it. We told her about a dog named Salty that used to spend an occasional weekend with us. Cindy adored this springer spaniel and to this day treasures the pictures of it. We wanted to get a similar dog for her. Patty told us that would be fine with her.

Patty moved into the house in January, with plans for Cindy to move back a few weeks later so Patty would have time to settle in. Once again, in an effort to give the family care provider as much comfort as possible, we gave Patty the largest bedroom, just as we had with Ann Marie. Previously, however, Cindy had taken the smallest bedroom, but this time we decided she should have the larger of the remaining two. There were no immediate plans for the smallest bedroom, although bringing in a second housemate was discussed.

Patty was an extremely busy person who, in addition to having a full-time job with the state, was also furthering her education. We found out later she also had a private counseling service, which she did out of the home. After she moved in, she wanted to move out a good deal of Cindy's furniture and move hers in. We explained to her again that we wanted this to be Cindy's home with her things. While we did not object to her bringing in some of her own things, we were concerned that Cindy continue to see and feel that this was her home. If a care provider moved out, we didn't want everything else to go also.

Patty also liked to have a good deal of time for herself and very often went away for a weekend or sometimes longer. During those times, her daughter and boyfriend, along with their young son, would stay with Cindy. For a short period of time, another woman also stayed in the house. This person was also found by the state to fill in some of the times when Patty was busy or away. For whatever reason, she and Patty did not hit it off, and Patty felt the woman was "giving off negative energy and invading her private space." Patty installed a lock on her bedroom door and kept it locked at all times. No one had a key, including me. That posed a problem because one time while she was away, there was a potential plumbing problem in her bathroom, and we couldn't gain access to attend to it. She was very upset when I asked later that she provide us or someone with the state a key to be used in case of emergency. As landlords who have responsibility for repairs, we didn't think that was an unreasonable request, but she felt it was an invasion of her privacy. The other woman only stayed a short time, so Patty relied heavily on her daughter for respite.

That June, Cindy "graduated" from high school. Because she was now twenty-one years old, she no longer could receive special education services. She was now a part of the adult service system and received twenty-five hours a week of day habilitation through another private not-for-profit agency. Cindy was no stranger to this agency as it used to be the Cerebral Palsy Center where Cindy was seen when she was younger. Other than the twenty-five hours a week of day programming, Cindy had no other activities or supports. Patty did very few activities with Cindy, so she ended up that summer not being very active. She was very bored and did a great deal of acting out.

Another person of Patty's choice moved in during that summer. Michelle was an interpreter for the deaf and knew Cindy from her summer program. We thought this would be a great addition to the house and would also give Patty some of the relief she wanted. Michelle was great with Cindy but was an extremely busy person and was also gone a great deal of the time. She also had a cat, and we were clear that we intended to get Cindy a dog.

CINDY GETS HER DOG

We found a springer spaniel that was very similar to Salty, and Cindy seemed thrilled and excited. Patty did not seem to share that enthusiasm. Getting the dog turned out to be a big mistake.

Very soon after Cindy got the dog, we started getting calls from the neighbors complaining about the barking. We had met them when we first bought the house, and they knew who we were and how to get a hold of us. Apparently, the dog spent a great deal of time in the backyard and barked all the time. Each time we received a call, we would in turn call Cindy's house and let them know. But the complaints did not stop. Our efforts to try and get the neighbors to speak directly to the ladies at Cindy's were unsuccessful, and the calls became even more frequent and angrier in nature. We made several visits to Cindy's house and drove by numerous times. It became apparent that the dog was indeed put out in the yard on a regular basis. Also, the cat apparently did not like the dog, so that made the situation worse because it was given priority over Cindy's dog.

One time we stopped by the house to see Cindy. The dog was in the backyard and was barking. Bob asked Patty if Cindy had fed her dog and was told she didn't think so. Bob went to help Cindy do that only to find out there was no dog food. When he asked Patty about it, she was not aware of it and said it was Cindy's dog, not hers. She could not tell us when the dog had last been fed. Bob went to the store and got some food and helped Cindy feed the dog. Judging from the way it ate, we assumed it had not been fed in a while. It was now obvious that we had to do something. We spoke to Patty about the dog and the complaints from the neighbors. She initially told us she was upset because Cindy herself did not choose the dog but later admitted that neither she nor Michelle wanted anything at all to do with it. I reminded her of our conversation regarding a dog before she moved in. She remembered the conversation and her agreement but told us she did not think it would ever be a reality. We found a home for the dog and said our goodbyes. I vowed there would be no more dogs.

CINDY IS BORED

There were some other problems at the house also. That summer was probably one of the nicest I have ever seen in our area. Cindy loves to be outdoors and always tans to a beautiful golden-bronze color. But this summer she was very pale, and it was obvious she was not getting out and doing things. We suspected that when Patty held her counseling sessions, she did so in her bedroom with the door closed, and Cindy was left unattended. When Patty's daughter and boyfriend were there when Patty was away, they attended to their son and not Cindy. One time I stopped over, and Cindy was in her bedroom in bed with the door closed at 7:00 in the evening, and she was clearly not happy about it. When I spoke to Patty about it, she told me she always put her "clients" in the group home to bed early. Cindy started to exhibit some aggressive behaviors again and had been breaking things. She had thrown something at her bedroom window and broke that, as well as the light in her closet, and several lamps had been thrown. I felt strongly she was doing that because she did not want to go to bed that early. And I felt she was bored because she was sitting around all day doing nothing.

One day I stopped late in the morning to drop something off. Patty was away, and her daughter was there with her boyfriend. Apparently, Cindy had become angry during breakfast and had thrown her cereal and orange juice, and it was all over the kitchen floor. As a result, Cindy was in her room by herself. Everyone else was in the living room watching a movie. It was almost lunchtime, and the mess from breakfast was still on the floor. It was a gorgeous warm summer day, and I suggested that perhaps Cindy could go for a walk or sit out on the deck. I told them I would be stopping by later to drop off something.

I returned later that afternoon and found Cindy sitting alone on the deck in a slight drizzle. I brought her back into the house and noticed that the mess from breakfast was still on the floor. I was livid and the next day called my case worker at the state and complained. Once again, the response from the state was "family care providers are very hard to find." Someone must have said something to Patty because she was very upset with me. Patty was so busy that she did nothing with Cindy. Cindy had no activities except for her limited day habilitation program and, judging from her behaviors, was bored to death. She was clearly telling us she was unhappy.

To top all of this off, there were also issues with the house. Michelle liked the windows open, and Patty liked the air conditioner on as it was a very warm summer. Their solution was to do both. I would come over and find windows open in many of the rooms, or the front door open and the air conditioning on. My efforts to explain that this only wore down the units and ran up the electric bill were for nothing, and I finally just put my foot down and threatened to shut the air conditioner off completely. By this time, I was being seen merely as an interfering parent who was totally demanding and unreasonable.

WE DO NOT MAKE THE SAME MISTAKE

The result of all this tension was that Patty decided to leave. While we do not think she was a bad person, we also think she never really understood what we were looking for. We wanted someone to be a part of Cindy's life. This was supposed to be more than just a job or a free place to live. It was supposed to be about Cindy and what she needed and wanted. Patty had a group home mindset and ran the house like a group home, with Cindy being in bed early every evening whether or not she was tired. The housemates were entertaining in the house but excluding Cindy. Cindy was not happy, and her behavior showed it.

Bob and I were very concerned that Cindy would end up back at home with us for another year. Because of that, after Patty gave her one-month, notice we refused to bring Cindy home or even take her anywhere. Our fear was that if Patty suddenly moved out before the date she had given and Cindy was in our care, the state would say the same they did before, and we would end up with Cindy back home for a long time again. So we came right out and told everyone that we would only visit Cindy in her home and only when Patty was present. It was so very difficult for us to take this stance, but we were so distrustful of the state we felt we had to do it.

Of course, one month is nowhere near enough time to find another provider or put things together, so when the time came for Patty to move out, Cindy was sent to a group home. When we went to her house to pack her clothes, Cindy cried and tried to get us to move out her kitchen table. We kept telling her that the table was going to stay and she would return, but she kept trying to push it toward the door. We tried to make her understand, but her heart was aching and so was ours. We felt like she was giving up and thought perhaps she felt that she had done something wrong. After all, it was the second time that the living situation in her house fell apart. It was heart-wrenching both for her and for us because we knew what would be happening to her.

Cindy bounced around from one state-run group home to another, even sleeping on the couch of one house. We made it very clear to everyone involved that she was their responsibility and we absolutely refused to bring her home permanently. We did go back on our commitment not to see her alone. If we hadn't, we would have had to spend a great deal of time in the group homes and we couldn't stand that. So we would pick her up and either bring her home for dinner or take her out somewhere. It was always so difficult to take her back as we knew she was not happy in these houses. We kept telling her we were working to get her back into her house but were having a difficult time making her understand that.

Some of the homes were better than others, but some were just awful. Once I went to pick up Cindy and found her sitting in the middle of the hallway of the house partially naked. This house had both male and female residents, as most do, and there was obviously no consideration given to people's privacy. When I entered the house, there would be several people sitting in the living room with no TV or radio on or no activity being done. People were just sitting and rocking. It was so difficult to see Cindy in that environment, and Bob could not bear to even walk into the place. He knew if he did, he would pack Cindy up and bring her home but he also knew the consequences of that action. We felt awful and terribly guilty.

Fortunately, Cindy ended up at a different house that was much better and she even had her own room. We still were not crazy about it as there were at least eight people living there, but the staff was nice and Cindy seemed to do a little better than she had at the others. Because of her situation, however, it was not a permanent placement, and she was still subject to being moved around. Cindy did not do well with change, and any move was difficult for her.

The next move was to a four-person house, all women. Cindy had some rough times in the beginning, with some acting out and destruction of property. Fortunately, the staff was very capable of handling it. One of the staff, Maxine, took a special liking to Cindy and did many activities with her outside the home. They developed a special relationship, and Cindy calmed down and for the most part did well in the house. She was there for several months, and during that time, Katy, Cindy's service coordinator at the time, visited her in the home. She mentioned to Maxine that they were searching for another family care provider, and Maxine expressed an interest.

NEW APPROACH, NEW PROVIDER

When Patty gave her notice, the folks at the DSO contacted the executive director of the NFP agency and asked if she was still interested in taking over supervision of the house. The ED, being the sharp lady that she is, told them they were not going to throw a hot potato in her lap. She knew the history of the past failures and made it clear that if they became involved, it would be done with careful thought and planning. The state agreed and we all started actively planning for her return to her house while Cindy was bounced around from house to house.

Everyone involved agreed that Cindy needed a great deal of support. One family care provider was not sufficient. It was agreed that a second person would be sought to live in the house and be paid to work with Cindy during those times the family care person was not there. This would allow the care provider to be able to have a job as well as maintain their outside activities.

MEDICAID WAIVER

The Medicaid Home and Community-Based Waiver program was in effect at this time and a proposed budget drawn up for the service. Because of Cindy's needs and the level of service required, the budget was considered an "outlier" and could not be approved by the local OMRDD office. Approval from the state offices in Albany, New York, was necessary. The paperwork was completed and sent through proper channels while we waited. The setup of Cindy's house was highly unusual, and there were only one or two in the entire state where families owned the home. Cindy was once again a pioneer and opening new doors for others. Family care typically was done in the family care provider's home, not the individual's who is being supported. Also, at that time it was extremely rare for someone with Cindy's needs to be living in their own home. So when the staff in the Division of Budget (DOB) in Albany saw the proposals before them, they could not understand what we were trying to do.

The process of getting a budget through Albany is tedious to begin with, but this situation added confusion and further gridlocks. The ED of the agency did everything she could to make them understand what we were trying to do, answering their barrage of questions. One day while in Albany, she went to visit the DOB and just sat and spoke with them, not asking anything from them but only telling them about Cindy and her life and what she had been through regarding her home.

I also did all that I could to help the process along by applying pressure where I could locally. I attended a conference sponsored by OMRDD and was told there were some important people there from DOB in Albany. The executive director of the agency pointed out the person I needed to talk to, and during the lunch break, I cornered him. I told him who I was, and he knew the last name and the proposal. I spoke to him about Cindy and how important it was to her that this go through so she could return to her home. I pushed him to help move it through the process and stressed to him the importance of doing so. He told me he would follow up on it upon his return and gave me his work number, telling me to call him if I hadn't heard from him within a week. Boy what a mistake he made giving me that number. He did call me the next week to say the proposal was in process and hopefully it would go through shortly. I asked if I could follow up with him if necessary and after hesitating he agreed. I ended up calling him about every two weeks or sometimes less, depending on what he told me. If he said it should be done in two weeks and there was no word in that time, I would call again. I was polite but persistent. The entire process of getting that budget approved and passed took almost a year. It was agonizing, but what resulted from it was that Cindy and her situation may have taught some people in Albany to look at people and their needs and not just numbers. Or maybe they just gave in to the squeaky wheel.

MAXINE

Once the budget passed and Maxine agreed to become the family care provider, the agency advertised for the additional live-in full-time position and found Virginia. Virginia would also live in the house rent-free and be paid for forty hours a week to be with Cindy. The additional position would be billed under the Waiver as Residential Habilitation. Now Cindy had 3 funding steams; family care, day habilitation, and residential habilitation, each service through a different agency. They each covered different times of the day. Virginia's time with Cindy would be those times when Maxine was at work or away from the home and Cindy was not in her day habilitation program. Maxine still worked at the same group home where Cindy lived, and her shift required her to be there overnight for three to four days at a time.

The day Cindy moved back into her home for the third time, she was so elated. She and Maxine eagerly packed up her things, and I picked them up. Maxine and Virginia both had already moved their things, and all of us as well as Katy were at the house to help Cindy unpack. This time we had decided to give Cindy the large bedroom, which had more privacy and its own bath. After all, this was her house and our previous efforts to give the nicest room to the family care provider seemed to be unappreciated. Maxine was quite content with that and she chose the smallest bedroom. Cindy was beaming from ear to ear and laughing. She was obviously very happy to be back in her own home. I took a picture of Cindy, Maxine, Virginia, and Katy, which showed how happy she was, and sent a copy of it with a note to the man in Albany. Someone told me much later it was the first time anyone had ever done that. They never had a face to go with a name.

Once Cindy settled into her new situation, she began to blossom. She became more independent and started doing more things for herself. Yes, there were still some rough times, but Maxine just worked through them. Maxine had a lot of experience in the field, and it was difficult for Cindy to get her flustered. Most things just rolled off Maxine's back, except when it came to relationships with others, which could be difficult. Despite that, she and Virginia got along well and lived together for almost a year before Virginia decided to move on.

I have always described Maxine as a free spirit of sorts. She marches to her own tune. Sometimes she would drive me nuts, but the bottom line was she cared deeply about Cindy and she had a good heart. Cindy lived with Maxine when she had to have an emergency dilation of her esophagus. Maxine thought Cindy had a stomach bug and kept her in bed and on liquids. When she no longer vomited and acted well, Maxine thought she was better. The two went out to breakfast the next morning and Cindy was eager to eat. When Cindy got sick again as soon as she ate, Maxine became concerned and called us. She brought her over to our house, and Bob knew instantly she was having trouble getting food down as even water at that point was difficult. I needed to take Cindy to the hospital, and Maxine offered to stay with Deb if Bob wanted to go also. Instead, however, Maxine took both Cindy and me. She stayed with us in the ER the entire time, lending support to not only Cindy but to me as well. I know it was uncomfortable for her but it was also obvious how much she cared about Cindy. Except for our parents' visit to the hospital when Cindy was first born, it was the only time that anyone was ever at the hospital to support us.

After Virginia moved out, Maxine's son's girlfriend moved in and took the full-time live-in position. Sherry and Maxine got along well, and the two of them took Cindy on several vacations, including one to Las Vegas. Maxine loved to travel and would usually take one or two trips a year, with one always in mid-winter. Cindy and Maxine developed a very special and close relationship, and they both loved to travel.

During the time Sherry lived with Cindy, she got a puppy without my knowledge or approval. After the experience with the other dog, I had set a rule of no pets. I was not happy about the puppy and should have demanded she get rid of it immediately. But housemates were difficult to find, and I was trying not to be difficult. It turned out I should have stuck to my guns because the puppy ended up being a big problem. Sherry did not know how to train a puppy and would not raise her voice or reprimand it. Consequently, the puppy peed and pooped all over the house, so much that the house began to smell. The puppy was a bone of contention between us until it was finally given away.

Maxine wanted to put an above-ground pool in the backyard, and together we did that. She purchased the pool, and we put in the electricity and landscaped around it. It turned out to be a wonderful thing for Cindy. She loves the water and spent hours in it when the weather was nice. Unfortunately, the next-door neighbors were not as crazy about it. The woman next door was furious and called us and demanded we put up a stockade fence. The yard was already fenced in with a metal fence that met the town's requirements, and I refused to put up another.

Part of the problem was that Maxine has a very large family and they very often all came over to use the pool. Maxine was a party person as was her family, and we started getting complaints from the neighbors about the noise. My efforts once again to try to get the neighbors to deal directly with the ladies that lived there were useless. The parties were not late, and the neighbors had no legal grounds, but it was obvious they had a point and I could understand their concern.

One time when Maxine and Cindy were away on a vacation, I got a call from a neighbor. They asked if I knew there was a pool party at the house during the day and early evening, which had become very loud. She also complained about the language being used. I went to the house and saw the trash can was filled with empty beer cans. I put a note on the door to the deck saying that under no circumstance was the pool to be used by anyone without my permission or the police would be called. Although Maxine's relatives did not like this decision, it was necessary. Fortunately, Maxine was a person I could talk to and reason with and explained these parties had to stop, as we were liable. We came to an agreement about the future use of the pool.

Sherry eventually moved out saying she was bored with the job and it was not challenging enough. Maureen, who was a person Maxine knew, moved in and took the full-time position. She was another party person and started taking Cindy to bars with her, which was of great concern to us. Maureen and Maxine would often get into arguments with each other, and I would be called to step in.

TROUBLE IN PARADISE

Maxine, Maureen, and Cindy, plus Maxine's sister, drove to Florida for a week's vacation. During that time, they took a day-long cruise. Maureen met a man and ended up ignoring Cindy when it was supposed to be her time with her. She and Maxine had some words over it. At the end of the cruise, Maureen left with the man she had just met, leaving Maxine, her sister, and Cindy to themselves. Maxine, who was known for her temper, was furious when Maureen finally returned to the hotel the next day, and Maxine would not let her back in the room. When Maureen demanded her belongings, Maxine refused. They apparently were packed in the same suitcase as the sister's things. Because her sister was not available to sort through it, Maxine refused to give anything to Maureen. Maxine never heard from Maureen after that. She and Cindy eventually left a couple of days later by themselves. When they got back home, Maureen's car was still in Cindy's garage. Maxine called all the agencies and informed them of what had happened. Maureen returned to town a week later thinking she would resume her place in the house. The agency, however, considered her to have abandoned Cindy and her job. Maureen was furious and blamed Maxine.

Shortly after, we were informed by the agency that Maureen had made a formal complaint about Maxine to the state authorities and there was going to be an investigation. Maureen accused Maxine of bringing men into their hotel room while Cindy was present, getting Cindy drunk on several occasions, and leaving her unattended in a car for hours at a time. The authorities did an investigation and found no evidence to support the accusations. I was interviewed as part of that and told the investigator that while I felt Maxine was not perfect by any means I felt strongly she would not do anything to jeopardize Cindy's well-being. The investigator tried to interview Maureen but she refused. We never saw her or heard from her again, and she left owing us several hundred dollars in back utilities. In addition, when she left on the vacation, she had possession of over $900 of Cindy's and our money, which was never recovered.

Although attempts were made to find another housemate, none was found and the position was partially filled by day staff. I think this was just fine with Maxine as she preferred to live alone with Cindy rather than have to deal with having a relationship with another housemate.

A TOUGH DECISION

Maxine lived with Cindy for almost five years and during that time their relationship grew even deeper. But eventually, Maxine decided it was time for her to move on. She hated winter weather, loved the sun and warmth, and the pressures and demands of her family were getting to her. So she decided she would move to the South. As was typical for Maxine, she had no definite plans, no job prospects, and no place to live. She merely quit her job of eleven years with the state and cashed in the savings she had accumulated. We were very concerned about Cindy and how she would react. Maxine gave us ample notice and agreed to stay until we found a replacement.

Maxine also had another solution to offer and that was for Cindy to move with her. She said she would go ahead and find a place and get settled and then Cindy could move down and live with her. She was serious and cared that much about Cindy. Because of that we did discuss it very briefly. As much as we were grateful for the relationship Maxine and Cindy shared, it just was not enough. Cindy would have no services in Florida, and we were unfamiliar with how to get them or the quality of them if she did have them. I only knew what I had heard from others in the field and that was they did not compare to New York State. We were also very concerned what would happen if things did not work out. If Cindy moved out of New York State, she would be out of the state's system. If she ended up moving back, even with us, she would have to start over from scratch getting services. She would drop to the bottom of a very long waiting list and nothing would be guaranteed. If we wanted her to live in her own home again, that process would have to begin all over again with new applications and approvals. It was a huge risk and there was no way we could take it.

There was also the emotional part of her moving. It would be much more difficult for us to see her and virtually impossible for us to communicate since Cindy does not read or write and the phone is useless to her. I could not just pick up the phone and talk to her to find out how she was and what was happening in her life. I would be completely dependent on other people for news. I explained to Maxine that there was no way I could not be actively involved in Cindy's life or at least be close by to deal with any issues that came up. As much as I had tried over the last few years to "cut the umbilical cord" and let go, this was just too much. Maxine understood that and said she would always remain Cindy's friend and Cindy would always be welcome to live with her.

We had heard that from so many others before that we did not count on it happening. People have good intentions but when they are no longer being paid or receiving something from the relationship, they usually lose touch. Cindy had many housemates and staff from various programs come and go, and many of them vowed to keep in touch. When they told us that, I always told them how hopeful we were that would happen and how important it would be to Cindy, but it never came to be. It would always be so hard on Cindy and ultimately on us to watch how upset she would be when people she cared about left her. It was as if she knew she would never see them despite what they said. I frequently tell people to be careful when they make promises because Cindy does not understand when they are broken.

Maxine turned out to be an exception to that. Although she lives in Florida, she did keep in touch for many years. She sent Cindy cards and included her picture so that Cindy knew they were from her. When in town she made a point to visit Cindy and spend some time with her. When Cindy traveled to Florida on vacation, Maxine met her wherever she was and they spent time alone together. Unfortunately, Cindy no longer hears from her.

Chapter 11

MORE PROBLEMS AND CHANGES CAUSE US TO RETHINK OUR PLAN

Catherine moved in with Cindy about a week before Maxine left to ease the transition. We were very concerned how Cindy would react and did not want her to think that because she was losing Maxine, she would lose her home also. That had been Cindy's experience in the past, but not this time. Catherine, who worked for the agency in one of their community residences, already knew Cindy from when Virginia lived with her so that was a definite advantage. She had a much more serious personality than Maxine but was also very experienced. Cindy did surprisingly well at first, taking the change with a good mood. We had a farewell party for Maxine and Cindy seemed very comfortable.

Unfortunately, the good mood did not last long, and shortly Cindy began to act out and destroy things again. We don't know if it was a delayed reaction to Maxine leaving or if it was the change of housemates or even something totally unrelated. That is what is so difficult about Cindy because sometimes you just never know what is going on with her. I suspect it was a feeling of insecurity and the change in personalities. Cindy needed to learn that Catherine was going to care for her just as Maxine had and that she would do things with her also. Fortunately,

Catherine was very good at dealing with Cindy's outbursts and handled them accordingly. I must give her credit as it took some time for Cindy to adjust and it was probably almost a year before she and Catherine developed a positive relationship.

CINDY TESTS EVERYONE

One of the things that must happen for Cindy to feel safe and secure with a housemate is to know that if she is sick, her housemate will be there to take care of her. Very often she will repeatedly ask for the doctor or dentist. It is sometimes difficult to know whether it is a real need or a test. One time with one of her housemates, Cindy kept asking for the dentist and pointing to a tooth. I told the person we needed to determine if this was real or not. The next day I got a call saying that Cindy must go to the dentist because she was in pain and the housemate was sure of it. She also had her sister who was a dental hygienist look at her tooth and she also thought there was a problem. I gave her the name and number of the dentist. Of course, there was nothing wrong with her tooth; it was merely Cindy testing her housemate, and the persistent signing for the doctor stopped after the visit.

Cindy can be very insistent. Sometimes she will ask to go to the doctor by repeatedly signing "doctor" to the point where she becomes angry. If someone signs "hurt" to her, she will sign "hurt" back. If you ask her if her left leg hurts, she will sign yes then sign over and over that her left leg hurts. It can be very difficult to redirect her attention. Then if you ask her if her right leg hurts, which is her artificial leg, she will also sign that that hurts and perseverate on that. When she does this, you can laugh it off and say it can't hurt, silly girl, and most times she will laugh also and drop it.

The other thing that must happen is for Cindy to know she will still get to go on her vacations. When she is with someone new, she will repeatedly sign vacation. She will be persistent to the point of agitation until she gets some kind of confirmation that she will go on a vacation. Usually what is the most effective is to show her on the calendar. Cindy will test in many ways but these two always seem to occur.

It is also important for people who work with Cindy to not be afraid of her. Sometimes that is difficult for some people when Cindy has grabbed them or scratched them. Cindy had a day habilitation worker who could not get beyond that. She worked with Cindy for many months, and during that time Cindy did not do well at all. Everyone involved with the residential part of Cindy's program tried to tell the day habilitation folks that this person was not a good match for Cindy. She was too much into Cindy's face, and Cindy did not like that. When Cindy started acting out, she became afraid of her and Cindy sensed it. Cindy will instantly take advantage of that and escalate her behaviors when she does not get what she wants. The relationship was not a good one, and Cindy's behaviors were jeopardizing her continuing in the program. We had many meetings and did much advocating to keep it intact. Things changed when the woman working with her left and someone else was assigned to take her place. It was difficult for the agency to find someone to work with Cindy because by now she had a reputation and many people were afraid of her. We had to work hard to overcome that.

PROGRAM CUTBACK

Cindy's original twenty-five hours of the day habilitation program was cut back to nineteen hours to give an hour a week for staff meeting and an hour a day for transportation and paperwork. Although I wasn't crazy about the cutback, I was still grateful she had a program and didn't have much of an argument. Twice after that in the years to follow, the agency would try to cut Cindy's hours. The focus of their program changed, and they ended up running two half-day programs because so many of their folks in the day habilitation program also worked in a job. Cindy's hours were adjusted from time to time to try to accommodate them, but when they tried to cut them further, I would not agree. Each time I would get into heated discussions with the program supervisor who would not give in. Then I would go over her head and write a letter to her supervisor, the head of the program. I had known this person for quite some time and have always found her to be reasonable. Both times she agreed not to cut Cindy's hours and reaffirmed their commitment to her.

Because of Catherine's work schedule and Cindy's limited program hours, a second housemate was needed. Samantha was sweet and easygoing, with no experience in the field, although she was willing to learn. In the beginning, she and Catherine seemed to hit it off. Over time, Cindy began to have some behavior issues and lashed out at Samantha and pulled her rearview mirror off her car. Samantha became concerned, refused to drive Cindy anywhere, and wanted some kind of support system. After many meetings, it was decided something would have to be done. At the same time, Cindy was also having the same problems at her day habilitation program, and they also wanted a plan of action.

A psychologist who consults with the agency was brought in to help. We had used him in the past, so he had some experience with Cindy. Many strategies for preventing Cindy from grabbing the driver while riding in the car were discussed, but no one solution was agreed upon. The suggestion was made that a special harness be purchased for the car. I was not crazy about this idea but agreed to look into it. Information was given to me, and Samantha and the people at day habilitation were pushing for it. The harness went on Cindy and then hooked onto a belt that was fastened in the car. It prevented her from leaning forward far enough to grab the driver. She still had freedom to move her arms and legs, but it restricted her forward movement. I reluctantly agreed to its use, and the psychologist wrote up very detailed and specific instructions in his plan. A cellphone was also purchased to be with Cindy at all times in case of an emergency. That part I thought was an excellent idea. Much to my surprise, Cindy didn't mind the harness and almost seemed to like the idea. Samantha was the only person who used it on a regular basis. Others such as Catherine or Anthony, her coordinator who filled in, merely sat Cindy in the backseat on the passenger side. We refused to use the harness when Cindy was with us. Some of the folks at the day habilitation program expressed interest in it and wanted us or the residential agency to purchase one for their use. Part of the harness was a fastener that fastened behind the seat, so transferring it from one vehicle to another was difficult. I flatly refused to pay for the harness because of my dislike for it, and the agency did not think they should have to pay for it either. Day habilitation never did purchase one, and eventually they did not see the need for it either. Samantha was the one who used it, and after she left, it was removed from Cindy's plan.

Cindy will sometimes go through periods where she has some undesirable behaviors, such as grabbing or scratching someone or ripping up something. She may go long periods of time without any of these and then have a burst of time when they occur frequently. How people react to these can play an important part in how long they last. People need to work to understand what is happening and how best to help Cindy through the difficult time. It can be a challenge, depending on the willingness of the people involved.

Cindy has also frequently had trouble sleeping at night. Even when she was at home, this was an issue and she never seemed to require a great deal of sleep. If awake at night, she can often get up and tear her closet apart or fling drawers out of a dresser. Over the years, various homeopathic solutions, such as melatonin or special teas, were tried but none were effective. The most effective solution is to make sure Cindy does not sleep late in the morning and is as active as possible during the day with no naps.

After obtaining the harness, Samantha returned to taking Cindy out but was still uneasy about being with her and did not do much with her. This of course only aggravated Cindy further. About this same time, the relationship between Samantha and Catherine deteriorated. Samantha had a boyfriend and although she had no tangible proof, she believed that he had cheated on her with Catherine. Samantha had met someone with supposed psychic powers who confirmed it. In addition, some things had happened between the three of them that had made Samantha suspicious. Catherine and Samantha's boyfriend of course denied anything was going on between them, but Samantha was convinced they were lying. Whether or not there was any truth to it will never be known nor is it anyone else's business. But what was our business was the drama and discord that resulted and the negative effect it was having on Cindy. It was not a good situation, and Samantha eventually gave her notice.

A SKILLED SIGNER — A GOOD THING, RIGHT?

It was a while before another housemate was identified. Several were interviewed and thought to be possibilities but they would back out or some problem would arise at the last minute. Eventually, Andrea moved into the house and took the full-time position.

Andrea was in her mid-twenties and a skilled signer, which was a definite asset. She said she intended to take the test to become an interpreter for the deaf. Catherine liked her and they got along well. I thought it would be a good match for Cindy because of her ties to the deaf community, but as soon as I saw her interacting with Cindy, I had some concerns. She was too strict with Cindy and too much in her face, which I knew Cindy did not like. She also had an attitude that she was an expert when it came to people who were deaf and was constantly telling others how to handle Cindy.

Shortly after she moved in, there was an agency dinner and Andrea brought Cindy to it. They sat with Bob, Deb, and me at a table I specifically picked out. I knew there was going to be a slide show, which Cindy would love, and I wanted to make sure she had a good seat. I saved the best viewing seats at the table for them. The executive director was narrating the slide show. I knew that night that Andrea would never pass the interpreter test. Although she was a skilled signer, she was a terrible interpreter, which is a very different thing. First, she positioned herself all wrong. She should have positioned herself so Cindy could see her and the screen but instead she sat on the side of Cindy and turned Cindy's chair partially away from the screen. When Cindy would look away from her to see the pictures, Andrea would physically turn Cindy's face back toward her. I have never seen an interpreter do that. In fact, in the many times that one has been hired for meetings for Cindy, if, during the meeting, Cindy should stop paying attention, the interpreter would merely stop signing until she resumed her attention. Andrea was just being a show-off. Also, at that dinner party, Andrea would not allow Cindy to have a glass of wine or even a soda as she felt it might cause some undesirable behaviors. There was some confusion about the setup in the restaurant, so there was no water available either. Our efforts to get Andrea to ease up on her restriction were unsuccessful. Bob wanted to just get something for Cindy despite the objections, but because Andrea was driving Cindy back and forth and ultimately responsible, we felt we shouldn't interfere. We did manage to get water to all the tables. I knew that evening that trouble was just around the corner and it was only a matter of time. I spoke with several people at the agency as well as Andrea to get her to change her ways but Andrea felt she knew best.

A couple of months later, Andrea took a week off to attend a training session at Gallaudet University in Washington, D.C. She would also be taking her test to become an interpreter and had talked about it with everyone. When she came back, I asked how it went and she told me she did not pass. She said she had fallen on some stairs early in the week and hurt her foot and that affected her test results. She did indeed have her foot bandaged and was wearing a soft boot-type cast. I was not surprised at all by the results but told her I understood her disappointment. The foot injury also ended up preventing Andrea from doing things with Cindy. She claimed it was too difficult for her with the cast.

CINDY IS TRYING TO TELL US SOMETHING, BUT NO ONE IS LISTENING

It was not too long before Cindy starting having some serious behavior problems with Andrea. Cindy was doing a great deal of grabbing at Andrea as well as other destructive behavior. Andrea claimed at one time that Cindy pushed her down but no one ever actually saw that happen, and I seriously doubted it did. We had several meetings, which included the consulting psychologist, to try to work things out. Cindy was very unhappy and was showing it. Her undesirable behaviors eventually carried over into her day habilitation program, and they were expressing great concern for Cindy. I continued to express my concern about Andrea and the way she interacted with Cindy, but housemates were so difficult to find I think the agency was reluctant to let her go. Even the people at Cindy's day habilitation program were expressing concern about Andrea.

One day I stopped by Cindy's house unannounced, which I seldom do. I usually call ahead. Andrea answered the door, and she was dressed to the nines saying she had a big date. She looked lovely, and I noted she was wearing spiked heels. I said nothing to her at the time except to wish her a good evening. The next day I was in the agency office for a meeting, and she also happened to be there. I noted she was back in her cast. I spoke to the coordinator and told him what I had seen the night before. I am not sure whether anything was said to her, but it wasn't long after that that Andrea gave her notice. Her reasons of course were that Cindy was too aggressive, and she couldn't deal with it anymore. It was true that Cindy was exhibiting some aggressive and inappropriate behavior, but as soon as Cindy was told Andrea was leaving, the behaviors immediately stopped.

After Andrea left, everyone involved with Cindy discussed her and Cindy's behaviors at one of Cindy's reviews. I pointed out to everyone that we all needed to pay more attention to what Cindy was trying to tell us. Her acting out was a definite form of communication in the only way she knew she could get our attention. Despite my reservations about Andrea, none of us picked up or acted upon the fact that Cindy was so unhappy. When we did not do anything about it, Cindy decided to take matters into her own hands. I am firmly convinced she purposely drove Andrea out. If we weren't going to get rid of her, then she would. Once again, she taught us a valuable lesson.

Cindy did not hear from Andrea again until many years later when she asked to take her out for a cup of coffee. They did spend some time together and coincidently Andrea also approached the agency about potential job openings and working with Cindy again. When this was mentioned at one of Cindy's meetings, I was totally shocked they were bringing this up. I reminded folks about our previous experience and objected to even the consideration of Andrea working with Cindy again. I told them I could not believe they were even talking about it. My statements were supported by the day habilitation staff who said they also felt it would be a terrible mistake. It was the last we heard of Andrea.

Another housemate was never found, although there were several interviewed and brought to the house. Some people in the agency felt at times Catherine purposely discouraged potential housemates because she did not want a roommate. Whether or not that was true we will never know, but Catherine did have her boyfriend stay over more and more to the point he just about lived there.

With the absence of a second housemate who was supposed to be full time, the agency provided the coverage and gave Catherine the support she needed to be able to stay there. Her regular full-time job required her to stay out very late or even overnight, and the agency filled in with relief staff whenever necessary. This was the big difference between this private not-for-profit and the state. It kept the house up and running and Cindy in it despite housemates coming and going.

ANOTHER BIG DECISION

Eventually after living with Cindy for almost six years, Catherine decided to move on and get a place of her own. We always knew the day would come, and fortunately she gave better than a year's notice. Cindy has not always accepted change well, and we were very worried how she would react.

The intent was to find two women who would share the house. One would be the family care provider, as was Catherine, and be overseen by the state. The other would be an employee of the NFP agency and in addition to living there would be paid for forty hours a week to work with Cindy. When we were going through this change, we were told that the state continued to look at this situation. They had been threatening for years to change the funding. The family care provider receives money from the state. Typically, a person with a disability lives in the family care provider's home, and the monthly allowance they receive is supposed to cover the cost of their room and board. The state loves this funding stream because they get the most for their money and it is usually the cheapest. At that time, family care providers typically got somewhere around $600 a month. In some cases, like Cindy's, they would also get a "difficulty of care rate," which is additional money based on the needs of the person living with them. In Cindy's case, the provider did get additional money, which was periodically reassessed. They also got allotments twice a year for clothing and vacations, as well as some other services. It is a great deal for the state. Granted, Cindy's house was not the typical family care model and was more expensive than most because of the additional staffing. However, if she were to live in a group home, it would probably be in a highly staffed house, which would be even more expensive.

When Cindy first moved into her own home, her residential services consisted of only the family care support from the state. Twice she was forced from her home because the care provider left. That is why the additional Residential Habilitation piece was added, to provide additional support as well as a safety net. This was put into place as a result of much advocacy on the part of the agency's executive director and me. With the additional support, Cindy always remained in her home despite the changes in housemates. The problem came when the state changed the way it bills family care. The difficulty of care rate was billed to Medicaid and so was Residential Habilitation. Although there were not two agencies billing for the same time, the state really did not want to do it. They eliminated all the other situations in the state like this except for Cindy's. Every time the issue came up, the agency would advocate on Cindy's behalf and it would remain.

So, when Catherine was leaving, the question came up again. I tried to get a commitment in writing from the authorities at the state to keep it intact. All I got was a verbal commitment. I stressed it was important that if they were going to make a change, it should be done then.

RETHINKING OUR PLAN

Our original idea of Deb being able to respite at Cindy's house never worked out. Most of the time, there were two housemates or sometimes boyfriends. It is a three-bedroom house and just not big enough. Also, the providers had their hands full dealing with just Cindy. When the state people kept telling us providers were hard to find, they were not wrong. Finding someone to live with both girls would be near impossible. The house would have to have rotating staff twenty-four hours a day, seven days a week. That in itself would pose all kinds of problems. We also realized that both girls living together was not the best thing for either of them. Although I believe they love each other, they are two very different people. When Cindy left home, Deb began to blossom. She became more outgoing and engaging. Part of the reason for that may be because she was in an inclusive classroom for the first time. It was an incredible experience that changed us all for the better in so many ways. And it also confirmed my belief Deb should continue that inclusion in her future living situation. So that left us with the question of where Deb would live when it was her time to move, which was approaching. We knew two things for certain: we did not want her to live in a group home, and we could not afford to buy another house. Because we purchased Cindy's home, it was titled in our names. We could not do that again. So, what do we do?

DEB HELPS CINDY

To plan for Deb, we assembled a group of people with expertise to help us. It consisted of a representative of a housing agency serving low-income people with disabilities, the director of the agency that was now involved with Cindy, our accountant, an attorney specializing in Medicaid law, people working with Deb, and of course Deb. We met on a regular basis, and each of us would leave with a task. The housing agency had a homeowner's program to assist individuals with purchasing a home. We really liked the idea of Deb also having her own home but did not know how we could do that. We had Deb apply for a mortgage at a bank and everything went along beautifully until it came time to sign the papers. Deb does not write and does not speak. We are Deb's legal guardians. The woman at the bank was clearly thrown by Deb's limitations. She did not know how to handle it or what to do. She said she would investigate it and get back to us but never did. This got us thinking about the safety of a house being in her name, so we consulted with the attorney. To protect her and her benefits, we decided a special needs trust would be set up to own the house. The trust would secure a mortgage, and Deb would pay rent to the trust. Her Social Security and subsidies through the Medicaid waiver would fund the rent. We paid for the cost of the trust and provided a small down payment for the house to keep the mortgage affordable for Deb. The housing agency secured first-time homeowner grants, as well as grants for the environmental modifications needed for wheelchair accessibility. And they helped secure a mortgage. They also oversaw all the needed renovations. This all took years, but Deb finally had her own home. Deb was present and involved in all of it. When Bob and I identified a house we thought would work, we showed it to Deb and she saw all that was being done. She was very excited. All the work would end up proving helpful to Cindy in the not-too-distant future.

A LOVELY FAMILY FOR CINDY

While looking for people to live with Cindy, our case worker at the state approached us about someone who was interested in the family care part. The only catch was that she had a husband and young child. The problem with that was it would eliminate the second live-in person. I was opposed to it at first but decided to at least meet the person.

Mary was a service coordinator who worked for the state and had over twenty years in the field. She came with very high recommendations, and after meeting her, I was impressed. This presented us with a very difficult decision. If Mary and her family moved in and something went wrong, there would be no back-up housemate to take over. We were eliminating the very safeguard we argued was so necessary. I was also concerned about their young son and how Cindy would react to him. Cindy had not lived with us for many years. The last few years she did live with us, she was clearly not happy. Bob and I were not sure how she would react to living in a family situation with a young child. At times when Cindy is frustrated, she will physically lash out at someone, either pinching or scratching them. My fear was that she would do that to the young boy, which would in turn cause his parents to leave. I kept pushing the state to assure me that if anything went wrong, they would support Cindy staying in her house. They continued to say they were committed to the situation.

Bob and I struggled with the decision for some time, not because we had any doubts about Mary and her family or their qualifications, but only about the stability of the house should anything go wrong. There was even division within the agency about which way we should go. Some felt a family was a great idea, while others thought that two unrelated housemates would be safer. If one housemate left, she would still have another. The decision was left to us.

By this time Deb had also moved into her own home. Coincidentally, we were going through some difficult times at Deb's house with a housemate that wasn't doing what she should be doing. It was very clear that finding good people was difficult. Finding two was even more difficult, and more often than not, they did not get along. We definitely had a quality person in Mary and would most likely not find another like her. So, we decided to put our fears aside and go for it. Because we had the luxury of time, which is very unusual, we had regular planning meetings to determine the best way to get Cindy through this. The forty-hour-per-week position would still be there, but it would not be a live-in position. It would be a full-time day position. Because of this, Catherine chose to move over to that position, which provided Cindy with some continuity. Although Catherine would not be living with

Cindy, she would be seeing her on a regular basis, and that made the transition much easier for Cindy.

Much to our delight, Cindy took the change like a champ, with virtually no problems. Mary and Jim are lovely people who made Cindy very much a part of their family. Cindy really enjoyed their son John, and I loved to watch them play together. Mary and Jim took excellent care of Cindy, paying very close attention to her health, particularly her weight problem. They made many sacrifices and they went on the same diet as Cindy to support her in her efforts. Cindy lost a good deal of the weight she gained while living with Catherine. Mary and Jim truly cared about Cindy and wanted what was best for her. Mary was not afraid to speak up for what she thought was right and best for Cindy even if it is not what people wanted to hear. Unfortunately, at times that was not welcomed by some agency staff.

Looking back, I now wonder why this decision was so difficult. But of course, I know Mary and Jim better now than when we first met. We had a good relationship, built on openness and honesty.

Cindy was happier than I had seen her in a very long time. She looked wonderful, partly because of some weight loss and partly I am sure because she was happy. She smiled and laughed a great deal. Mary and Jim worked on her being more independent, and Cindy was doing just that. Cindy enjoyed John, and the two of them got along beautifully. I think Cindy had found what she loved growing up and what we can no longer give her, a large family. Bob and I had very few family members still alive. Mary and Jim and John made Cindy very much a part of their family and she loved it. They are lovely people who I hoped would stay with Cindy for a long time.

IT IS ABOUT CINDY

As with everything else in our lives, things do not always go smoothly. Although Cindy was doing very well, there were numerous problems. Mary and Jim were not happy with the staff and the way they were doing things. This caused a great deal of stress for them and us as well. There was a great deal of turmoil. Efforts to resolve the issues were unsuccessful. Unfortunately, the focus was no longer on Cindy, but despite that, she was doing very well. Mary had indicated to me many times her unhappiness with the situation, particularly with the agency providing the staff. While I admit they did not always handle things right, I was not ready to change to another agency. It just is not that easy. Cindy and I had a long history with this agency. They were committed to keeping Cindy in her home no matter what. Other agencies would not do that. And I was not convinced that changing agencies would solve all the problems.

I tried to do everything I could to make things right. I reminded everyone that this situation was about Cindy. I told them I was convinced that if Cindy could speak, she would tell us she wanted everyone to get along for her sake. She did not want to lose anybody. It was an unfortunate example of how people lose sight of the main focus, that is Cindy, and get caught up in their own agendas and personalities. Many meetings were held but it still was not enough. After living with Cindy for two years, Mary and Jim decided they could no longer do it. They agreed to stay until another provider was identified, provided they could minimize their involvement with all the agencies. Eventually, they felt they could not wait any longer and gave a little over a month's notice. I was very worried about how Cindy would take this change. It was clear she did not want them to leave.

THE BIG DECISION

Because Mary was moving out, we were faced with new decisions. The state would no longer allow both family care and Residential Habilitation. We were faced with tough choices. We had many meetings with people from the state and the NFP agency talking about funding and how best to give Cindy what she needed. One of my options would have been to keep the house as a family care home with only the state involved. We would lose the NFP's direct involvement. I must admit the woman from the state I was working closely with was wonderful and extremely supportive. It was very different from my previous experience. She assured me of their commitment to Cindy, and I did not doubt her sincerity. But people come and go, and my decision did not require a great deal of time to make. Bob and I felt strongly we could never again put our child totally in the hands of the state. Our past experiences were too painful.

We had a few other choices, but of course nothing is ever perfect. In the end, we opted to eliminate the state involvement and stay entirely with the NFP agency. They had stood by Cindy for many years, and people there knew her and believed in her. I shared their philosophy and believed their commitment to the people they support. Her services were somewhat redesigned and worked out better for Bob and me. We were able to transfer ownership of the house to a special needs trust for Cindy, the same as we had just done for Deb. This would ensure it would be hers always and still protect her benefits. We had set up testamentary special needs trusts many years before to make sure when we passed that our assets would be available to the girls and their benefits protected.

With the house in a trust, we would now get some financial relief from the housing expenses. Cindy would now qualify for housing support she was not able to get previously and she also would pay rent to the trust. The rent covers the housing expenses. A search was started for new housemates.

CINDY STAYS IN HER HOME

During all these planning meetings, Cindy was still unaware that she was losing the people she cared about so much. We have learned over the years it is best sometimes not to tell Cindy things too far in advance. I was terribly worried how she would react. I knew it was doubtful we would find housemates before Mary and Jim left so the house would be staffed. The agency was keeping its promise to Cindy and would make sure she stayed in her house.

I was afraid Cindy would react badly and start her destructive behaviors again. I was afraid she would view it personally and feel she had failed. Others also worried about her. So everyone, including Mary and Jim, the agency, and us, did all we could to make the transition as easy as possible on her. I was exhausted from worry and the lack of sleep. But as she has done so many times before, Cindy surprised us. After the initial disappointment of finding out, she handled things beautifully; she did incredibly well and was still happy. She has seen Mary, Jim, and John since they moved out and thoroughly enjoyed that. She adjusted nicely to the addition of new staff.

Fortunately, her full-time staff continued with her and took on a new sense of responsibility. The agency, recognizing the difficulty of the transition, arranged for Catherine, her former housemate, to spend some time with her. Everyone worked together for Cindy's best interests. The situation wasn't the best, and there were lots of changes. But once again, Cindy surprised us and showed all of us how far she has come. She did well, and it was obvious how much she has grown. I have learned that no living situation, whether individualized or not, is perfect. There will always be problems and constant changes.

During the next several years, there were many changes in the staff, and housemates came and went. But the constant is that Cindy remained in her home. She is very proud of her home and takes great interest in it. She frequently lets us know what she would like done, such as painting, new flooring, or appliances, and she even wants new siding. She will often point out something that needs to be fixed. When our long-time contractor does work at her house, Cindy will often gesture to him about things she thinks needs his attention. She will point to an area and sign "paint" or a light fixture and sign "fix." She really does love her home.

Chapter 12

HOW ARE THE GIRLS DOING NOW?

There have been many changes in the system of services. Now services are provided through Self Direction. This new funding is supposed to give greater control to the individual or their family. It can be complicated and is always changing. It also puts greater responsibility on individuals and families. They are required to provide their own backup and must stay within a budget. It lessens the burden on the state.

This is a story about Cindy. But so much of who Bob and I have become has also been shaped by Deb. She too has taught us many things. Deb is very different than Cindy. Cindy had many medical issues at birth; Deb did not. Cindy cannot hear but Deb can. Cindy's eyesight is keen; Deb does not see well. Cindy can walk; Deb uses a wheelchair. Deb has her own story.

DEB

In 2002, at the age of twenty-two, Deb moved into her own home. She adjusted beautifully, much better than her parents. In many ways, we did not want her to go, but due to some health issues of mine, her care was becoming too difficult for me. And we wanted to make sure she was set for the future.

Deb likes a calm environment, free of commotion and drama. She loves music and has an extensive CD collection. She has a happy personality and is almost always upbeat. Although she is nonverbal, she often makes what we call her hoot and holler, telling us she is happy or excited. And she can hum "Twinkle Twinkle" perfectly. She wakes up happy almost every day. She is smart, has a beautiful smile, and an infectious laugh that can brighten the dullest of days. She is known for her fashion style of bright colors and different hair accessories.

When Deb moved into her home, we experienced many of the same issues with finding the right housemates and staff. But Deb loves her home and especially enjoys her beautiful deck in the nice weather.

In 2013, we were fortunate to find a wonderful woman to live with Deb. Kim is a kind, giving, and loving person who takes excellent care of Deb, as well as her home. They have developed a beautiful relationship, and it is obvious how much they care about each other. Kim understands Deb and her needs and recognizes her many strengths, often when others do not. She does not hesitate to advocate for what Deb needs and always has her best interest at heart. We have open and honest communication between us. Kim also helps with appointments when I am unable to do so. Like Cindy, Deb also receives supports during the day. But Kim is the glue that keeps it all together and she does that well. She is truly remarkable and irreplaceable.

Deb and Kim will soon celebrate ten years together, and we are so grateful to have her in our lives. We consider her family. Kim brings so much to Deb's life. She is understanding and patient with ongoing staffing issues, and she gives so much of herself. While Deb has always seemed happy, now she seems more so than ever. Deb is thriving.

CINDY

In 2011, we found Cheryl, a new housemate, now called a live-in caregiver, for Cindy. Support is provided to her by staff, now called mentors, who take Cindy out into the community. Mentors have come and gone. There has been funding changes and an agency change. But throughout it all, Cheryl has stayed.

Cheryl is a wonderful woman who is easygoing, caring, and compassionate. She and Cindy have developed a beautiful, loving relationship. She takes exceptionally good care of Cindy even as her medical needs increase again as she ages. Cindy has been treated for many years for obsessive compulsive disorder (OCD) and has also developed chronic pulmonary issues. The pulmonary issues can be very problematic as she has frequent bouts of intense coughing and is easily prone to pneumonia. Cheryl deals with all of this and rarely complains.

In 2020, when I was diagnosed with a life-threatening illness and required numerous treatments and surgery, Cheryl took over oversight and management of Cindy's medical. She continues to do most of it. She has become a terrific advocate for Cindy and always has her best interests at the forefront. We have always maintained good communication between us. As Bob is in his 80s and I am in my late 70s, this is a tremendous comfort to us. Quite frankly, I do not know what we would do without her.

Cheryl has a good deal of energy, which is good because Cindy keeps her on the go constantly. The two of them shop, eat out, go to shows and various activities, and travel together. They visit Cheryl's relatives and host parties for them. Cindy loves big parties. Cheryl has a large family, and they have all made Cindy very much a part of it. She has given Cindy what she has always loved and what we no longer have, lots of relatives.

Cheryl also helps Cindy to pursue her love of arts and crafts. And to Cindy's and our delight, she takes excellent care of the house.

Cindy's behaviors can still be challenging at times, but Cheryl deals with them beautifully. She has incredible patience. As much as Bob and I love Cindy, we recognize how difficult it can be to live with her and marvel at how Cheryl does it. Few people would. We certainly no longer could.

We consider Cheryl a part of our family. You only have to watch the two of them together to know how much they care about each other. And Cindy is truly happy. This really is a life-sharing relationship. After more than twelve years, Cheryl and Cindy continue to live together. It does not get any better than this. There is not a day that goes by that we are not incredibly grateful to have Cheryl in our lives. She is truly an extraordinary woman.

We are so fortunate to have not one but two beautiful, wonderful women to be with each of our girls. I could not wish for anything better. I do not know what I would do without them. I give thanks every day for both of them. We are truly blessed.

CINDY'S IMPACT

Cindy has faced many challenges medically, educationally, and in day-to-day life. There will always be hurdles to overcome. But I have also watched Cindy and seen first-hand how very far she has come. Change is not easy for anyone, but Cindy now accepts those changes much easier. She is a remarkable example of the success one can achieve when offered opportunities, when allowed to take risks, and yes, when allowed to fail. Being a parent of a child with a disability is indeed a challenge. It is a constant struggle, and just when you think you have everything going the right way, something changes. It is constant advocacy and it will be done as long as I can physically do it. I will take it to my grave. Cindy has come so far and grown so much and continues to thrive. Yes, there are good days and bad, ups and downs, but overall, her star is shining brighter than ever.

Cindy changed our lives dramatically. Yes, in many ways, life has been difficult but she also changed us for the better and shaped Bob and me into the people we are today. Besides loving her as any parent would, her father and I have a tremendous respect for her and all she has accomplished. She gave us strength and purpose. She helped to mend a difficult relationship and brought our family closer together. She is responsible for me discovering abilities and courage I never knew I had. Because of Cindy, I learned how to advocate and now use that knowledge to help others; in return I receive many benefits. Because of Cindy, Deb got the help she needed much earlier and continues to benefit from all Cindy's experiences.

Cindy also inspired other people. Some decided to enter the field of special education because of their experiences with Cindy. Others became more sensitive, caring, and tolerant because they knew Cindy.

Cindy taught many medical personnel that they did not always have the right answers. She showed them the impact of their mistakes and hopefully made them more conscious of possibilities. She also taught them to listen better, not just with their ears but with their eyes and their hearts. Communication comes in many forms.

Cindy has also taught many professionals to respect parents more and give more credence to their opinion. Cindy proved that sometimes the so-called experts are anything but that. No matter what their claims, in the end, Cindy would have the final say. Sometimes that happened at tremendous cost to her and us as well. But we believe because of all Cindy has been through, some professionals have learned to be a little more cautious. They may not jump to conclusions that can do harm. And they may not throw all their training out the window without a careful and objective analysis of a situation.

Cindy paved the way for others with disabilities. Transportation in school is now easier because of her. She set legal precedent for special educational services within regular public-school settings. She was a pioneer in creative housing for people with disabilities.

When people take the time to truly know Cindy, they soon realize what a remarkable woman she has become. They are often touched by her and genuinely like and admire her. They consider her a friend. They often tell me she inspires and motivates them. I understand that because she has done that for me since the day she was born. Cindy was not supposed to live. She was supposed to be a "vegetable." We were told she would never walk. We were told she would never live independently. She has proven so many people wrong and she has accomplished so much. She has overcome more obstacles and adversities than any person should have to. Yes, she has had some help along the way, and the supports will be ongoing. But it is truly her and all she has gone through that has changed so many lives.

When I think about a "crusader," I think of someone who fights to make a change. I think of an advocate, a champion for a cause. I think of someone who puts their heart and soul into making something better, not just for themselves but for others as well. Cindy has done all those things and has done so with a passion and intensity rarely seen. She has done so with strength and courage and incredible perseverance. Her effort is endless and untiring. In my mind, she truly is a crusader, who has never uttered a single word.

FINAL THOUGHTS AND ACKNOWLEDGEMENTS

Raising two children with disabilities is not easy. It can be challenging and exhausting but also very rewarding. I have benefited in many ways. This story, although sometimes difficult, I hope will be inspiring to others. Even though a person has a disability, they still have so much to offer.

There have been many people along the way, too numerous to mention. But a few stand out for me. Some may have passed on, or I have lost contact.

The four parents, Kitty, Ellen, Paula, and Mike, who helped with the transportation issue set me on the path to becoming an advocate for others. I never have forgotten what they did and their impact. I have kept my promise to give back and that has brought me many rewards.

Others, both parent and professional, were role models and advisors. People like Bernice, Hillary, Jo, Bob and Sue, Pat, Kim to name a few. Sandee taught me so much about advocacy and navigating the system.

There have been many friends as well as professionals who have supported us along the way. We are forever grateful.

Debbie, we have known each other for over thirty years. You are a dear friend, a wonderful advocate for our girls, and an important part of our lives. Thanks for caring so much. You have our eternal gratitude.

To Mark and Cora, thanks for having our backs.

To all the mentors, our broker Michelle, and all the other support people along the way, thank you. We could not have done it without you.

Thanks to Kim and Cheryl, two of the most extraordinary women one could meet. For over ten years, you have given so much to each of our girls. We could not find better caretakers. You both are such loving, caring, unselfish people. You are our girls' family as well as ours. They love you and so do we. I cannot tell you enough how grateful we are to have you in our lives. I give thanks every day.

Scott, you are my brother, mentor, confidant, advisor, problem solver, cheerleader, and so much more. I love you and could not ask for a better brother. Thank you for always being there for me.

And finally, to Bob, you are a wonderful husband and father. Anything we have accomplished was in large part because of you. Thank you for your support the last fifty-five years. And thank you for allowing me to tell this story. I love you so much.

Printed in the USA
CPSIA information can be obtained
at www.ICGtesting.com
LVHW091230011123
762283LV00001B/8